SPECIAL NEEDS IN ORDINARY SCHOOLS
General Editor: Peter Mittler

Children with Speech and Language
Difficulties

Special Needs in Ordinary Schools

General editor: Peter Mittler
Associate editors: James Hogg, Peter Pumfrey, Tessa Roberts, Colin Robson
Honorary advisory board: Neville Bennett, Marion Blythman, George Cooke, John Fish, Ken Jones, Sylvia Phillips, Klaus Wedell, Phillip Williams

Titles in this series

Children with Speech and Language Difficulties

Alec Webster and Christine McConnell

Cassell

Cassell Educational Limited
Artillery House
Artillery Row
London SW1P 1RT

British Library Cataloguing in Publication Data

Webster, Alec
  Children with speech and language
  difficulties.—(Special needs in
  ordinary schools)
  1. Children—Language   2. Language
  disorders in children   3. Remedial teaching
  4. Speech therapy in children
  I. Title   II. McConnell, Christine
  III. Series
  371.94'4   LB1139.L3

ISBN: 0 – 304 – 31378 – 5

Typeset by Activity Ltd., Salisbury, Wilts.
Printed and bound in Great Britain by Biddles Ltd.,
Guildford and King's Lynn

Last digit is print no. 9 8 7 6 5 4 3 2 1

Contents

Foreword: Towards education for all

This series aims to support teachers as they respond to the challenge they face in meeting the needs of all children in their school, particularly those identified as having special educational needs.

Although there have been many useful publications in the field of special educational needs during the last decade, the distinguishing feature of the present series of volumes lies in their concern with specific areas of the curriculum in primary and secondary schools. We have tried to produce a series of conceptually coherent and professionally relevant books, each of which is concerned with ways in which children with varying levels of ability and motivation can be taught together. The books draw on the experience of practising teachers, teacher trainers and researchers and seek to provide practical guidelines on ways in which specific areas of the curriculum can be made more accessible to all children. The volumes provide many examples of curriculum adaptation, classroom activities, teacher–child interactions, as well as the mobilisation of resources inside and outside the school.

The series is organised largely in terms of age and subject groupings, but three 'overview' volumes have been prepared in order to provide an account of some major current issues and developments. Seamus Hegarty's *Meeting Special Needs in Ordinary Schools* gives an introduction to the field of special needs as a whole, whilst Sheila Wolfendale's *Primary Schools and Special Needs* and John Sayer's *Secondary Schools for All?* address issues more specifically concerned with primary and secondary schools respectively. We hope that curriculum specialists will find essential background and contextual material in these overview volumes.

In addition, a section of this series will be concerned with examples of obstacles to learning. All of these specific special needs can be seen on a continuum ranging from mild to severe, or from temporary and transient to long-standing or permanent. These include difficulties in learning or in adjustment and behaviour, as well as problems resulting largely from sensory or physical impairments or from difficulties of communication from whatever cause. We hope that teachers will consult the volumes in this section for guidance on working with children with specific difficulties.

The series aims to make a modest 'distance learning' contribution to meeting the needs of teachers working with the whole range of pupils with special educational needs by offering a set of resource materials relating to specific areas of the primary and secondary curriculum and by suggesting ways in which learning obstacles, whatever their origin, can be identified and addressed.

We hope that these materials will not only be used for private study but be subjected to critical scrutiny by school-based inservice groups sharing common curricular interests and by staff of institutions of higher education concerned with both special needs teaching and specific curriculum areas. The series has been planned to provide a resource for LEA advisers, specialist teachers from all sectors of the education service, educational psychologists, and teacher working parties. We hope that the books will provide a stimulus for dialogue and serve as catalysts for improved practice.

It is our hope that parents will also be encouraged to read about new ideas in teaching children with special needs so that they can be in a better position to work in partnership with teachers on the basis of an informed and critical understanding of current difficulties and developments. The goal of 'Education for All' can only be reached if we succeed in developing a working partnership between teachers, pupils, parents, and the community at large.

ELEMENTS OF A WHOLE-SCHOOL APPROACH

Meeting special educational needs in ordinary schools is much more than a process of opening school doors to admit children previously placed in special schools. It involves a radical re-examination of what all schools have to offer all children. Our efforts will be judged in the long term by our success with children who are already in ordinary schools but whose needs are not being met, for whatever reason.

The additional challenge of achieving full educational as well as social integration for children now in special schools needs to be seen in the wider context of a major reappraisal of what ordinary schools have to offer the pupils already in them. The debate about integration of handicapped and disabled children in ordinary schools should not be allowed to overshadow the movement for curriculum reform in the schools themselves. If successful, this could promote the fuller integration of the children already in the schools.

If this is the aim of current policy, as it is of this series of unit texts, we have to begin by examining ways in which schools and school policies can themselves be a major element in children's difficulties.

Can schools cause special needs?

Traditionally, we have looked for causes of learning difficulty in the child. Children have been subjected to tests and investigations by doctors, psychologists and teachers with the aim of pin-pointing the nature of their problem and in the hope that this might lead to specific programmes of teaching and intervention. We less frequently ask ourselves whether what and how we teach and the way in which we organise and manage our schools could themselves be a major cause of children's difficulties. Questions concerned with access to the curriculum lie at the heart of any whole-school policy. What factors limit the access of certain children to the curriculum? What modifications are necessary to ensure fuller curriculum access? Are there areas of the curriculum from which some children are excluded? Is this because they are thought 'unlikely to be able to benefit'? And even if they are physically present, do they find particular lessons or activities inaccessible because textbooks or worksheets demand a level of literacy and comprehension which effectively prevents access? Are there tasks in which children partly or wholly fail to understand the teacher's language? Are some teaching styles inappropriate for individual children?

Is it possible that some learning difficulties arise from the ways in which schools are organised and managed? For example, what messages are we conveying when we separate some children from others? How does the language we use to describe certain children reflect our own values and assumptions? How do schools transmit value judgements about children who succeed and those who do not? In the days when there was talk of comprehensive schools being 'grammar schools for all', what hope was there for children who were experiencing significant learning difficulties? And even today, what messages are we transmitting to children and their peers when we exclude them from participation in some school activities? How many children with special needs will be entered for the new General Certificate of Secondary Education examinations? How many have taken or will take part in Technical and Vocational Education Initiative schemes?

The argument here is not that all children should have access to all aspects of the curriculum. Rather it is a plea for the individualisation of learning opportunities for all children. This requires a broad curriculum with a rich choice of learning opportunities designed to suit the very wide range of individual needs.

Curriculum reform

The last decade has seen an increasingly interventionist approach by Her Majesty's Inspectors of Education, by officials of the Department of Education and Science and by individual Secretaries of State. The Great Debate, allegedly beginning in 1976, led to a flood of curriculum guidelines from the centre. The garden is secret no longer. Whilst Britain is far from the centrally imposed curriculum found in some other countries, government is increasingly insisting that schools must reflect certain key areas of experience for all pupils, and in particular those concerned with the world of work (sic), with science and technology, and with economic awareness. These priorities are also reflected in the prescriptions for teacher education laid down with an increasing degree of firmness from the centre.

There are indications that a major reappraisal of curriculum content and access is already under way and seems to be well supported by teachers. Perhaps the best known and most recent examples can be found in the series of ILEA reports concerned with secondary, primary and special education, known as the Hargreaves, Thomas and Fish Reports (ILEA, 1984, 1985a, 1985b). In particular, the Hargreaves Report envisaged a radical reform of the secondary curriculum, based to some extent on his book *Challenge for the Comprehensive School* (Hargreaves, 1982). This envisages a major shift of emphasis from the 'cognitive–academic' curriculum of many secondary schools towards one emphasising more personal involvement by pupils in selecting their own patterns of study from a wider range of choice. If the proposals in these reports were to be even partially implemented, pupils with special needs would stand to benefit from such a wholesale review of the curriculum of the school as a whole.

Pupils with special needs also stand to benefit from other developments in mainstream education. These include new approaches to records of achievement, particularly 'profiling', and a greater emphasis on criterion-referenced assessment. What about the new training initiatives for school leavers and the 14–19 age group in general? Certainly, the pronouncements of the Manpower Services Commission emphasise a policy of provision for all, and have made specific arrangements for young people with special needs, including those with disabilities. In the last analysis, society and its institutions will be judged by their success in preparing the majority of young people to make an effective and valued contribution to the community as a whole.

A CLIMATE OF CHANGE

Despite the very real and sometimes overwhelming difficulties faced by schools and teachers as a result of underfunding and professional unrest, there are encouraging signs of change and reform which, if successful, could have a significant impact not only on children with special needs but on all children. Some of these are briefly mentioned below.

First, we are more aware of the need to confront issues concerned with civil rights and equal opportunities. All professionals concerned with human services are being asked to examine their own attitudes and practices and to question the extent to which these might unwittingly or even deliberately discriminate unfairly against some sections of the population.

We are more conscious than ever of the need to take positive steps to promote the access of girls and women to full educational opportunities. We have a similar concern for members of ethnic and religious groups who have been, and still are, victims of discrimination and restricted opportunities for participation in society and its institutions. It is no accident that the title of the Swann Report on children from ethnic minorities was *Education for All*. This, too, is the theme of the present series and the underlying aim of the movement to meet the whole range of special needs in ordinary schools.

Special needs and social disadvantages

Problems of poverty and disadvantage are common in families of children with special needs already in ordinary schools. The probability of socially disadvantaged children being identified as having special needs is very much greater than for other children. Children with special needs are therefore doubly vulnerable to underestimation of their abilities – first, because of their family and social backgrounds and, second, because of their low achievements. A recent large-scale study of special needs provision in junior schools suggests that, although teachers' attitudes to low-achieving children are broadly positive, they are pessimistic about the ability of such children to derive much benefit from increased special needs provision (Croll and Moses, 1985).

Partnership with parents

The Croll and Moses survey of junior school practice confirms that teachers still tend to attribute many children's difficulties to adverse home circumstances. How many times have we heard comments along the lines of 'What can you expect from a child from that kind of family?' Is this not a form of stereotyping at least as damaging as racist and sexual attitudes?

Partnership with parents of socially disadvantaged children thus presents a very different challenge from that portrayed in the many reports of successful practice in some special schools. Nevertheless, the challenge can be and is being met. Paul Widlake's recent books (1984, 1985) give the lie to the oft-expressed view that some parents are 'not interested in their child's education'. Widlake documents project after project in which teachers and parents have worked well together. Many of these projects have involved teachers visiting homes rather than parents attending school meetings. There is also now ample research to show that children whose parents listen to them reading at home tend to read better and to enjoy reading more than other children (Topping and Wolfendale, 1985; see also Sheila Wolfendale's *Primary Schools and Special Needs*, in the present series).

Support in the classroom

If teachers in ordinary schools are to identify and meet the whole range of special needs, including those of children currently in special schools, they are entitled to support. Above all, this must come from the head teacher and from the senior staff of the school; from any special needs specialists or teams already in the school; from members of the new advisory and support services, as well as from educational psychologists, social workers and any health professionals who may be involved.

This support can take many forms. In the past, support meant removing the child for considerable periods of time into the care of remedial teachers either on the school staff or coming in from outside. Withdrawal now tends to be discouraged, partly because it is thought to be another form of segregation within the ordinary school, and therefore in danger of isolating and stigmatising children, and partly because it deprives children of access to lessons and activities available to other children.

We can think of the presence of the specialist teacher as being on a continuum of visibility. A 'high-profile' specialist may sit alongside a pupil with special needs, providing direct assistance and support in participating in activities being followed by the rest of the class. A 'low-profile' specialist may join with a colleague in what is in effect a team-teaching situation, perhaps spending a little more time with individuals or groups with special needs. An even lower profile is provided by teachers who may not set foot in the classroom at all but who may spend considerable periods of time in discussion with colleagues on ways in which the curriculum can be made more accessible to all the children in the class, including the least able. Such discussions may involve an examination of textbooks and other reading assignments for readability, conceptual difficulty and relevance of content, as well as issues concerned with the presentation of the material, language modes and complexity used to explain what is required, and the use of different approaches to teacher–pupil dialogue.

IMPLICATIONS FOR TEACHER TRAINING

Issues of training are raised by the authors of the three overview works in this series but permeate all the volumes concerned with specific areas of the curriculum or specific areas of special needs.

The scale and complexity of changes taking place in the field of special needs and the necessary transformation of the teacher-training curriculum imply an agenda for teacher training that is nothing less than retraining and supporting every teacher in the country in working with pupils with special needs.

Whether or not the readers of these books are or will be experiencing a training course, or whether their training consists only of the reading of one or more of the books in this series, it may be useful to conclude by highlighting a number of challenges facing teachers and teacher trainers in the coming decades.

1. We are all out of date in relation to the challenges that we face in our work.
2. Training in isolation achieves very little. Training must be seen as part of a wider programme of change and development of the institution as a whole.
3. Each LEA, each school and each agency needs to develop a strategic approach to staff development, involving detailed identification of training and development needs with the staff as a whole and with each individual member of staff.
4. There must be a commitment by management to enable the staff member to try to implement ideas and methods learned on the course.
5. This implies a corresponding commitment by the training institutions to prepare the student to become an agent of change.
6. There is more to training than attending courses. Much can be learned simply by visiting other schools, seeing teachers and other professionals at work in different settings and exchanging ideas and experiences. Many valuable training experiences can be arranged within a single school or agency,

or by a group of teachers from different schools meeting regularly to carry out an agreed task.

7. There is now no shortage of books, periodicals, videos and audio-visual aids concerned with the field of special needs. Every school should therefore have a small staff library which can be used as a resource by staff and parents. We hope that the present series of unit texts will make a useful contribution to such a library.

The publishers and I would like to thank the many people – too numerous to mention – who have helped to create this series. In particular we would like to thank the Associate Editors, James Hogg, Peter Pumfrey, Tessa Roberts and Colin Robson, for their active advice and guidance; the Honorary Advisory Board, Neville Bennett, Marion Blythman, George Cooke, John Fish, Ken Jones, Sylvia Phillips, Klaus Wedell and Phillip Williams, for their comments and suggestions; and the teachers, teacher trainers and special needs advisers who took part in our information surveys.

Professor Peter Mittler   University of Manchester
                                                  January 1987

REFERENCES

Croll, P. and Moses, D. (1985) *One in Five: The Assessment and Incidence of Special Educational Needs*. London: Routledge & Kegan Paul.

Hargreaves, D. (1982) *Challenge for the Comprehensive School*. London: Routledge & Kegan Paul.

Inner London Education Authority (1984) *Improving Secondary Education*. London: ILEA (The Hargreaves Report).

Inner London Education Authority (1985a) *Improving Primary Schools*. London: ILEA (The Thomas Report).

Inner London Education Authority (1985b) *Educational Opportunities for All?* London: ILEA (The Fish Report).

Topping, K. and Wolfendale, S. (eds.) (1985) *Parental Involvement in Children's Reading*. Beckenham: Croom Helm.

Widlake, P. (1984) *How to Reach the Hard to Teach*. Milton Keynes: Open University Press.

Widlake, P. (1985) *Reducing Educational Disadvantage*. London: Routledge & Kegan Paul.

Acknowledgements

So many colleagues and friends have given their help in the course of writing this book that it would be impossible to acknowledge them all. However, we would particularly like to thank the speech therapists, psychologists, doctors and teachers who have shared our professional concerns in Berkshire, in endeavouring to meet the needs of children with speech and language difficulties.

For the best part of a decade we have been fortunate in working with the Audiology Unit at the Royal Berkshire Hospital and with the Linguistics Department of Reading University. In reading and commenting on the manuscript, Corinne Haynes, Margaret Parker and Patricia Scanlon have helped shape our thinking.

We owe a special debt to David Crystal for his advice. Both Peter Mittler and James Hogg gave us much constructive criticism and encouragement. Ronnie Vickery patiently and expertly typed the various drafts of the manuscript, and to her we are much indebted. Our respective families gave us an abundance of inspiration and evidence, but the parents and children with whom we continue to work in partnership have helped us most of all.

Alec Webster   Reading 1986
Christine McConnell

1

Introduction: Language and special needs

Language is normally such an integral part of every social and intellectual experience that it seems a contradiction to discuss it as a subject apart. In this book we shall be looking at aspects of children's play, social relationships, behaviour, and emotional maturity, as well as their thinking and reasoning. In reading and writing too, children learn for the same purposes, and use the same skills, demanded by listening and speaking. It follows that any problems in communication will inevitably be reflected in their wider school achievements. So, whilst this is a book about speech and language difficulties, these issues are not discussed in isolation. It seems to us to reflect misguided policy whenever 'language work' appears as a separate item on the class timetable. This is not to say that some children do not require abundant opportunities to use and develop language skills.

On the other hand, it is because language holds such a critical and complex position in development, that we need clear and simple models to understand it. In this book we shall be addressing the ordinary class teacher who may have a special interest in language, but not necessarily any special qualifications or experience. We have tried to make the theoretical issues as accessible as possible, and to provide a framework for thinking about language which will allow teachers to develop their own insights. The book should answer many of the questions teachers often ask about how communication develops, how and why it goes wrong, and, when a child has special difficulties, what the teacher needs to do differently.

Wherever possible the text has been illustrated with practical examples taken from our own contacts with children, families, and schools. The book will have succeeded in its aims if it enables teachers to understand, identify, and take steps towards helping children with communication problems. That can only be achieved by accepting that children's difficulties relate, not only to themselves and their 'disabilities', but also to the environments in which they live, play, and learn.

The underlying theme of this book is that language is not a

'subject' which can be taught separately or directly. Furthermore, we hold in high regard the natural and spontaneous skills of the majority of parents as they interact with their young children at home, particularly in relation to the development of language. Consequently, we feel that professionals should be careful about devaluing or changing the behaviour of parents, in the (perhaps mistaken) belief that experts know best and have all the answers. Without doubt, in our opinion the school's best efforts are directed at optimising conditions for learning in line with the view that children are generally more effective learners than we are teachers; and that is perhaps the hardest lesson of all.

HOW MANY CHILDREN HAVE A LANGUAGE DIFFICULTY?

Child: 'Him no got none Peter.'
Adult: 'What? Tell me again.'
Child: 'Peter, Peter.'
Adult: 'What about Peter?'
Child: 'Him apple, no.'

Faced with a new experience children may use language to describe, compare the unfamiliar with the known, explain events, or simply convey feelings to someone else. Language enables children to think out and shape their perceptions of the world, and to express their reactions to it. At one level language can be seen as a vehicle: a means of representing information in a message. At another level language is the means by which a child achieves and maintains social contact with other people. In the example given above, the child's particular difficulties in using language disturb most of the functions we have mentioned: how the child classifies and communicates his experience, and the social interaction he sustains with another. Indeed, this child's limited powers of expression immediately cause some uneasiness: 'What is the child trying to say?'.

It is not always easy to decide what constitutes a language problem and when to express concern about a particular child. The reason for this is simple: all children are different in the way they begin to develop speech and language, and in their rates of progress. It has already been stressed that a communication difficulty cannot be discussed as an isolated aspect of a child's overall development. Nor do children fall neatly into categories so that they can be readily counted. Language difficulties cover a very wide range of factors and are probably best approached by way of descriptive continua, which help us to observe the different aspects of a child's language competence.

At one end of the scale a significant language difficulty encompasses the child with a slight pronunciation problem, such as a lisp, a speech hesitancy, or mild stutter. Even relatively minor speech problems cause anxiety and sap confidence, particularly if they persist into school age. At the opposite extreme, children known to have a sensory handicap, such as a severe hearing loss, may experience marked communication problems. These might include the pronunciation of speech sounds; acquisition of words, phrases, and sentences; together with the use of language as a means to learn. Some children are simply slow to develop along normal lines, but eventually catch up with their peers. Their speech and language skills emerge later than is usual, and such children may be difficult to understand and use immature sentence patterns in school.

Other children have much more fundamental problems in organising and understanding language, and these may still be evident in adulthood. Language, in all its forms, appears to hold little meaning. The languages of symbolic play, of pictures, and of the written word all seem as difficult to grasp as speech itself. Children with a serious and persisting difficulty specific to language development, without any underlying factors such as limited ability, hearing loss or physical handicap, are relatively rare. When severe and specific language problems arise, the child is at risk of a wide range of social, emotional, and learning consequences. However, it is no easy task to predict how the course of development will proceed. Parents are sometimes advised that an infant who has no words by the age of 18 months, or is not using short sentences by three years, may be in need of special help. Without wishing to seem complacent about these early warning signs, several children are known to the authors who had not made a start on talking by four years, but rapidly became 'experts' in their first year at nursery. Some perfectly ordinary toddlers later develop problems as language is used in different ways in school, for example, in reading and writing.

The field of language disability is thus characterised by diversity. In developing normal communication most children call on good senses, motor skills, intelligence, and a nurturing social environment. Disturb any one dimension and the pattern of language growth may also be affected. So too, since many aspects of normal psychological development are heavily interwoven with language skills, the child who is unable to communicate will be hindered in making full use of learning opportunities. Such a diversity of underlying contributory factors and resultant features is the main reason why there have been few exact estimates of the number of children with a language difficulty in the population at large.

Several large-scale studies have been completed in the United Kingdom, in which the incidence and prevalence of a wide range of handicapping conditions in childhood, including speech and language, have been estimated. (Incidence refers to the number of children with a particular difficulty being added to a population, for example, during the course of a year. Prevalence refers to the proportion of people in a given population exhibiting a particular condition.) The National Child Development Study followed the progress of all the children born in Britain in one week of March 1958. After the first follow-up, when the children were seven years of age, information was published on the developmental progress of some 15,000 children (Davie, Butler and Goldstein, 1972). One of many aspects assessed included the children's speech. Medical officers judged 14 per cent of children to have speech difficulties, whilst teachers identified nearly 11 per cent. Boys were much more likely to be identified than girls, as were children from the lower socio-economic groups. The second follow-up at age 11 years suggested higher figures than this, depending on the method of assessment used (Calnan and Richardson, 1976). Using a speech test, doctors' and teachers' ratings and the views of parents, altogether some 24.6 per cent of the population of children were identified, by one method or another, as having speech difficulties. This study highlights the need to specify very clearly what is meant by the term 'speech difficulty' and how it is going to be assessed. It is quite obvious from the little overlap between people's assessments that they do not always agree on what constitutes a speech problem.

In a study of families living in Newcastle (Morley, 1965), some 19 per cent of children aged three years nine months had communication difficulties. These included delays in speech, stammering and articulation problems. Ten per cent could not make themselves understood at three years nine months, five per cent at four years nine months and 0.7 per cent at six years six months. When researchers have screened children for the more serious, specific language difficulties, much lower figures have been reported. Surveys in Edinburgh and Aberdeen (Ingram, 1963) estimated that children thought to be of average intelligence, with only a few single words at three years and very limited connected speech at five years, numbered less than one per thousand. Figures from the Isle of Wight study (Rutter, Tizard, and Whitmore, 1970) give a similar figure of 0.8 per thousand with severe language problems at school age. On the other hand, in the Isle of Wight study more than half of the children thought to be of limited intelligence continued to have articulation defects and poor language throughout school age. Similarly, children identified as having reading problems tended to be late in talking, and to have poor language, as well as articulation defects.

Taken as a whole, these early surveys show that there is a high prevalence of speech problems throughout early infancy. Some five per cent of children enter school unable to make themselves understood, whilst more severe and specific language problems arise in about one per 1000 children. Twice as many boys as girls are affected. Speech and language difficulties are highly likely to be present alongside other handicapping conditions. (See also, Rutter and Martin, 1972.)

Of the more recent studies, Fundudis, Kolvin, and Garside (1979) followed up all the children in Newcastle who were not using three words together by the age of three years. Four per cent of children failed this simple speech screen. About one in five of this group later showed serious language, intellectual or physical handicaps. A survey of Dunedin children (Silva, McGee, and Williams, 1983) found 8.4 per cent of three-year-old children had language problems, through the administration of a battery of tests, including the Reynell Developmental Language Scales. Richman, Stevenson, and Graham (1982), working in Waltham Forest, found 3.1 per cent of three-year-olds to have a moderate delay in speech, 2.3 per cent with more severe delays, and 0.57 per cent considered to have specific speech problems. In a more intensive study of smaller groups of children, Bax, Hart, and Jenkins (1983) assessed all the pre-school children in two areas of Central London. Using an informal method children's speech was rated as being 'normal', 'possibly abnormal', or 'definitely abnormal'. At two years some 17 per cent were thought to have possible problems, whilst 5 per cent definitely did. At three years about 12 per cent were thought to have possible problems, whilst 8 per cent definitely did. By the age of four and a half years, 7 per cent were felt tentatively to be abnormal, and 5 per cent confidently so.

What should we make of this array of figures? It is quite apparent that a considerable number of young children do not develop speech and language at the normally-expected rate, with about five per cent entering school with communication difficulties, and a much smaller percentage experiencing persistent and specific problems. So there is a fair degree of consensus with the earlier surveys. Where all these studies vary is in the terms by which speech and language difficulties are both defined and measured. Some screening procedures are not very sensitive and perhaps pick out children who do not have any problems. Other tests correctly identify children, but there may then be disagreements about the degree of difficulty which should concern us. Clearly, tests which pick up very mild degrees of difficulty will identify greater numbers of children. It is for reasons such as these that studies differ in the kinds of language problems identified, and in the numbers of children who are estimated to have special needs. Perhaps the most interesting question is how far a child's failure on an early screening test can predict difficulties later on in childhood, but that is an issue which has been little investigated.

The Quirk Report (DES, 1972) on speech therapy services in the United Kingdom suggested that about three per cent of pre-school children, and about two per cent of school-aged children, have problems so severe as to require speech therapy. Of children placed in special schools 40 per cent were thought to need speech therapy help. Speech therapists are regularly involved in working with other special groups, such as the hearing-impaired, autistic children, and the emotionally disturbed. Many children whose major difficulties bring them into contact with psychologists, social workers, or remedial teachers, may also have language problems. In what he feels to be a conservative estimate Crystal (1984) suggests that around ten per cent of all children, both pre-school and school-age, have a language handicap which is serious enough to pose problems for themselves and their adult caretakers. If this figure is accepted, the implication for teachers working in ordinary schools is that approximately two or three children in every class can be expected to have a language difficulty of a greater or lesser degree.

THE URGE TO COMMUNICATE

Why do children need to learn language? The capacity most children have for using symbols to code events and to represent ideas about the world, makes it *possible* for children to learn language. In other words, ideas about events in the world are carried by language, not events themselves. However, the basic impetus for language learning is the urge to communicate. The child has a need to find out about the objects and events in the environment, to know what others think and say, and to pass on feelings and views. The child is motivated, then, to discover more about the world through communication. We can summarise this by saying there are two basic explanations for language development: firstly, skill in symbolic thinking; secondly, the human drive for complex social interaction with those who share the environment, in order to learn more about it.

This line of thinking has some important underlying assumptions. For example, we assume that language must have a social context in which the speaker is trying to communicate and share meaning with a listener. Also, children and adults do not talk about *nothing*: both must have something purposeful to say. Language is usually experienced by the child in an important, meaningful situation, particularly at home. Communication, then, has real purpose and intention and revolves around things which matter to the participants. It is all too easy when we analyse extracts from children's spoken language, and, more importantly, when we think about trying to *teach* language in school, to forget that normal communication is tied to a significant and purposeful social context.

The second underlying assumption concerns the *active* drive the child brings to language encounters to make sense of the system. The child is sometimes described as a scientist, actively discovering and testing out the environment. There is an urgent momentum to piece together the rules of language because of its functional importance. Psycholinguists interested in the psychology of language suggest that 'As language develops, it becomes a tool of the child's striving to derive meaning from his world' (Smith, Goodman, and Meredith, 1976, page 12). Later on in this book we shall be looking at the implication for teachers of this view in which the child takes the central role in discovering and generating the rules of language through *using* language. Fortunately, adults seem especially tuned to the language-learning needs of young children. We can see how proficient adults are in the conversation strategies they adopt with infants, in giving just the right amount of feedback, and in intuitively paraphrasing and expanding what the child says. However, the adult's role in this process is as facilitator, not teacher. Adults provide the stimulus and opportunity for linguistic interaction to take place. But it is the child's own task to organise and make sense of language experience. Much of this book, then, is concerned with the conditions which seem to be optimal for children as they strive to master the rules of the adult language system in which they are immersed.

THE FUNCTION OF LANGUAGE

Studies by researchers such as Bruner (1975), Schaffer (1977) and Trevarthen (1979) have shown that the foundations for language interaction are laid in very early infancy. From the outset mothers read meaning in their child's responses, actions, and moods, and claim to understand everything that the baby means. In the first few weeks mothers establish patterns of smiling, touching, looking, and vocalising. Talk accompanies everything that the child does in the social context of feeding, dressing, bathing, and changing. Both adult and child share experiences in which gestures and tone of voice, as well as words, are used to signal intentions and coming events, and to register feelings. The baby in a cot who cries because of being startled by an unfamiliar noise will evoke a response which rescues it from discomfort. Contrast this with the sounds which register delight as the mother comes home from work, and which evoke a mutual pleasure of greeting.

So a child's urge to socialise is motivated and supported by the adult's immediate responsiveness. The first games played by mothers with their babies, such as 'Peek-a-boo', 'Five little mice came out to play', or 'This little piggy went to market', have a significant function. They are the first shared dialogues in which the child takes part; the first 'turn-taking' exchanges, when initially the mother, and then the baby responds. Later on the child uses these conventions in recognising when to speak and when to give someone else a turn. It is also in these early, non-verbal exchanges that the infant learns to use eye contact to sustain interaction, and by looking away, to discontinue it. One other very important building block is the child's ability to follow the mother's line of gaze, so that when the mother names an object, the infant's visual experience is tied to the linguistic.

The linguist Halliday (1975) recorded the utterances of his young son Nigel, from 9 to 18 months of age. Halliday asked the question 'What does the child learn to do by means of language?' He looked at language as a form of interaction between the child and other people through which behaviour is regulated. Language has a function: to manipulate, change or control. It is a means to an end. In Halliday's terms, then, the child learns what language is through what it *does*. According to Halliday, there are seven distinct functions which language serves for the very young child.

1. Instrumental

In this function language is used by the child to express material needs: 'More drink', 'I want a go'. Even before the child has any recognisable words, babbled sounds and gestures may convey to the adult that the child wants a particular toy, or is hungry.

2. Regulatory

Children make the discovery that they can try to control the behaviour of others through language, in just the same way as others try to control them. 'Come for lunch'; 'Lift me up'; 'Go home now'.

3. Interactional

This is the 'me and you' function, used specifically to interact socially with important people and including meanings such as 'It's nice to see you'; 'Where are you?'; 'You came my house'.

4. Personal

Here the child expresses feelings about, reactions to, and interests in things in the environment. Halliday calls this the 'Here I come' function of language: 'I'm fed up'; 'You've got new hair'; 'All sticky now'.

5. Heuristic

The heuristic, or learning function is used by the child to explore and find out. It includes demands for names of things: 'What's that?' and later develops into a wide variety of questioning, such as 'When?'; 'Why?'; and 'Where?' This is the means by which the child categorises and discovers the world; 'Where's your daddy?'; 'That hot?'

6. Imaginative

Pretend play, story, and make believe, and moving into a world of fantasy are the imaginative function of language. Through this the child creates, predicts and explores events outside the 'here and now'. It enables the child, through role play, to learn about the real-life situations on which fantasy is based; 'My baby is ... '; 'Cos she really was ... '; 'might be ... '.

7. Informative

The final, and probably latest, use of language is to inform. Passing on information dominates adult's use of language. It is also true that most adults *believe* the major function of language to be the conveying of information to someone who requires it; the 'Let me tell you this' function: 'He's on the swing'; 'It's like my Mummy's only hers is broken'; 'We went to Hayling and we saw a smash!'

Halliday's survey of the different functions of language in early childhood underlines some very important points. What the child knows about language and how it is put to use may be very different from what the adult thinks, does and believes. In the early stages very little of what the child says is 'informative'. Children learning language use this function least of all, and not at all before the age of about two years. And yet the image which predominates in the adult's thinking about language is that its major use is to convey information. Halliday says that the informative function is 'The only purely intrinsic function ... definable solely by reference to language' (Halliday, 1975, page 21). In other words, for the young child, language serves a wide range of functions, including social, manipulative, interactional as well as informative purposes. These issues are of great importance when we come to consider the learning context, such as the school. Language is most efficiently acquired in a functional context where it is put to use. The child is not a passive recipient of language and the initial power of language for the child is in the social action it serves.

THE IMPORTANCE OF LANGUAGE IN SCHOOL

When teachers are asked to consider what their general aims are in working with children, they usually agree on the proper concerns of education:

- Achieving independence
- Developing as a person
- Self-discipline
- Enjoyment and understanding of others
- Ability to think clearly
- Practical skills
- Literacy and numeracy
- Knowledge of the world
- Realising individual potential for living and working
- Preparation for adult life

All these are aspects teachers would consider appropriate goals for every child. No distinction is made between ordinary children and those with a special learning difficulty. As the Warnock Report (DES, 1978) has recently pointed out, whilst some children may require more help in achieving these goals, nevertheless the aims of education remain the same for all. If we take a close look at what teachers are working towards and the methods and materials at their disposal, the fine grain of teaching is patterned by language. Language forms an inextricable part of *everything* that goes on in the classroom.

So, when the child reaches school age we can identify another set of functions served by language. Through talking children communicate their problems and fears and can be helped to a better understanding of their feelings and reactions to others. Adults can explain other people's points of view and why certain behaviour is good or unacceptable, together with the underlying reasons for any rules or restrictions on behaviour. The child learns, through discussion, the principles behind approved ways of behaving; and as Tough says (1977, page 10), 'Children may come to regulate their own behaviour by referring to the same principles.' Language, here, is the means by which the teacher expresses the social mores of the school, to foster an atmosphere of trust, respect and responsibility.

Children also use language to direct and organise themselves, and to shape their thinking. Through dialogue with the teacher the child's urge to enquire, question and discover, is encouraged. We can set out these important learning processes as follows:

- Describing events in experience
- Categorising events by relating new to old
- Outlining a sequence of incidents
- Extracting important concepts
- Connecting one idea to another
- Analysing a process
- Recognising cause and effect
- Making judgements by weighing evidence
- Predicting what might happen next

Language is not only a vehicle for projecting oneself into the feelings and behaviour of others; it is also a means of creating fantasy and imaginary worlds. Verbal reasoning is closely enmeshed with intellectual growth: how we reflect, analyse and interpret our perceptions.

Later on the child applies a knowledge of what spoken language is and does to encounters with written language in books. For most children, and with good reason, the written word provides a 'window into knowledge', a limitless aspect upon society's intellectual and cultural heritage. Reading and writing extend the child's ability to handle language into the 'disembedded' or reflective mode, and to an awareness of aesthetic aspects of the written word. In other words, the child has access to a form of language which outstrips the capacity of speech to handle complex, creative or abstract ideas.

A glance at any of the recent publications on the primary school curriculum, such as *A Language for Life* (DES, 1975) and the national primary school survey (DES, 1978), leaves little doubt about the central significance accorded to language in school. Whilst some people might disagree over the selection and emphasis, and whether schools do actually foster these skills, we give here what the Bullock Report (DES, 1975, page 67) suggests is an 'effective record' of the child's language experience in school:

- Reporting on present and recalled experiences
- Collaborating towards agreed ends
- Projecting into the future; anticipating and predicting
- Projecting and comparing possible alternatives
- Perceiving causal and dependent relationships
- Giving explanations of how and why things happen
- Expressing and recognising tentativeness

- Dealing with problems in the imagination and seeing possible solutions
- Creating experiences through the use of imagination
- Justifying behaviour
- Reflecting on feelings, their own and other people's

LANGUAGE DIFFICULTIES

Given the central importance of language in early childhood and in school, it comes as no surprise that the child who experiences difficulties in acquiring and using language will have tremendous obstacles to surmount in order to learn. This will, of course, be felt initially in the social interactions between child and adult care-takers, which often become emotionally charged and fraught where there is a problem of communication. We know, too, that children who come to school with a fluent, sophisticated grasp of spoken language make better all-round progress and achieve literacy quickly. Conversely, children who are considered to be very immature and restricted in their spoken-language abilities, and who are unable to absorb through listening for any length of time, will be seriously held back in school. Quite simply, the expanding needs of the child in learning and thinking are closely dependent on a growingly sophisticated language framework. We should not underestimate the deep and pervasive influence of language difficulties upon the child's development.

A child may be described as having a language difficulty when, at a time at which other children have succeeded, the use of sounds, words or phrases has not been mastered. The child is unable to encode knowledge and experience effectively. Similarly, such a child still has to learn how to use language to converse, enquire, manipulate and enjoy social interaction with others. It will be helpful, at this point, to introduce in some detail the main terms used to define and depict the child whose language fails to develop normally.

Global Developmental Delay

When we say that children are delayed in their development we mean that the skills the child has are well below the level expected for a child of a given age. A child with *global developmental delay* might lag behind the peer group in many ways, such as motor and co-ordination skills, social independence, emotional maturity, thinking and reasoning, together with understanding and using speech. An important aspect of global developmental delay is that

the child's skills emerge in the usual sequence, although progress
may be slow.

*Julie, a little girl with Down's syndrome, showed a wide range of
developmental delays at the chronological age of four years. She was a
heavily built child who had bottom-shuffled for a long time in order to
get about and still did not walk alone, manage stairs, run or jump
well. These 'large muscle' skills are normally mastered by two years.
Julie still wore nappies but was beginning to help take her clothes off
and dress herself, and could sit herself at the dinner table and eat with
a spoon and fork. Her social-independence skills were felt to be around
a two and a half year level. Julie loved hearing stories read and
appeared to understand a lot of what was said to her, but had only a
handful of words herself such as 'Mama', 'car', and 'hot'. Most
children have a vocabulary of 20 words well before the age of two
years. In her drawing, and play with toys and materials, Julie was not
yet at the stage where her play was representative: she could not draw a
man or pretend to feed her doll. Again, one would normally expect
these stages to have been reached much earlier.*

Knowing the sequence of development in different skill areas and
the ages at which various skills can usually be observed gives us the
criteria against which Julie's development can be contrasted. Many,
but not all, Down's syndrome children are slow to develop. Not all
of a globally delayed child's skills may be equally far 'behind'. In
chapter 3 we shall be looking at studies which have reported that, in
Down's children, language functioning could well be at a lower
level than other areas. Developmental delay may also occur in
children without any known or associated handicapping condition.
Such children may be helped at home, or in nursery, by a special
programme designed to foster a wide range of independence, motor
and language skills. In school these children may benefit from a
curriculum modified for children with learning difficulties, small
teaching groups and a slower-paced environment with more
individual help. Any special help devoted to speech and language
would be an integral part of an overall learning programme.

Developmental Language Delay

We can distinguish between a developmental delay affecting a wide
spectrum of skills in childhood, and a more specific difficulty arising
mainly in the area of the child's language growth. Such a delay
might be mild or severe, but, importantly, when the child's
language does appear, it follows the normal sequence and pattern.
The question might be raised at this point: What do we mean by

language? Of course there are many aspects of a child's language which could be involved, including speech sounds, knowledge of words, and use of grammar. Later in this chapter we shall be outlining some of the continua which are often used to describe language difficulties. In chapter 2 a fairly thorough account is given of the major dimensions used to describe normal language development and which therefore shape our thinking about how language development can go wrong. For the moment, however, some examples are presented of commonly occurring language problems.

Some children have difficulties in just one area of their language growth. A good example of that is the child who, although using a wide range of vocabulary and sentence structures, has immature *phonology* or speech sounds. The speech characteristics of a very young child persist much later into childhood than expected.

As a four-year old in nursery, Karen's speech gave these examples (transcribed in brackets):

> Oo go oo gagi on
> (You've got your glasses on)
> Me like boo n odwin bet
> (Me like blue and orange best)
> My dad go fit n tiptop
> (My dad's gone to the fish and chip shop)
> Ooperma fydown
> (Superman flies down)

The underlying reason for this may have to do with a weakness in auditory perception, so that the child does not spontaneously self-correct her own speech in line with the speech models around her. Both good hearing and good perceptual skills – ability to make sense of and respond to sounds – are required of the child. A speech therapist may be able to help such a child by careful assessment of the developmental level as a base-line against which progress could be measured. The therapist would suggest appropriate activities and opportunities for building up skills of auditory perception and discrimination. For example, a simple picture game would help Karen discover for herself the contrasts of meaning between ' cup of *tea*' and 'a door *key*'.

Another, but perhaps more serious, developmental delay in language affects children's ability to express themselves. Such children may have fairly mature phonology and appropriate vocabulary. They may understand a great deal communicated to them. The difficulty arises when children attempt to put words together in sentence structures to express what they mean.

Stephen at eight years was a quiet, non-communicative child who seldom returned answers in class, and when he did these would be just one or two words like a telegram message: 'Where my book?'; 'What that boy do?' Stephen did not know how words changed to indicate tenses, plurals or possessives: 'David Daddy did have two car.' When he wrote words down Stephen would start a sentence but not finish it, and he stuck closely to a few phrases which he knew: 'and I got ... ', 'The man went ... ' He seemed unable to put any of his own ideas onto paper, even from very recent and exciting experiences. On many occasions the sentence patterns of early infant reading books obviously overwhelmed him.

What kind of help might this child require? Since almost every area of his functioning in school was affected, Stephen required a small teaching group with a lot of individual help. He needed a teacher with the time and skill to help him expand on his ideas by introducing new vocabulary at the right moment and by providing ample opportunity for using and reinforcing rules for changing tenses, plurals and so on. Reading material would have to be chosen carefully or newly written around his interests, allowing him to build up to more complex sentence structures. In fact Stephen spent some of his time in a special language unit in an ordinary school, and the work of such a unit is described more fully in chapter 5.

Finally, a developmental language delay might involve *all* areas of linguistic skill, including sounds, words, sentence patterns and the general comprehension of language.

Christine, at almost five years, had a long history of middle ear infections which had resulted in a conductive hearing loss. Although the hearing loss was only mild it came and went persistently, and began to affect her development. In nursery, Christine was visually aware, having a good idea of colour matching and sorting. She noticed small details in pictures and was quick to understand the nursery routine.

However, Christine seemed totally unaware when instructions were given out, took little part in singing, word games or storytime, and was slow to grasp concepts of time and quantity. When adults talked about things outside of the immediate visible context, she lost interest. Her sentences were short and limited in content: 'My Mummy come soon', 'My Andrew got birthday', and she never enjoyed any 'to and fro' chatter with other children. Christine's speech was difficult to understand because of the unusual sound patterns: 'lelilant' (elephant), and word sequences: 'not you come my house.'

This child required very careful monitoring of her fluctuating hearing so that appropriate medical treatment could be given quickly. Adults needed to be aware of Christine's listening difficulties, especially in noisy conditions. In quiet situations, when her attention had first been gained and lots of non-verbal clues (such as gestures, facial expression, pictures, toys) given, Christine was able to understand much more of what was said to her and, in turn, began to use more language herself. The kind of strategies which adults can use with children who have listening difficulties are outlined in some detail in chapter 5.

Language Disorder

Not only is there delay in the language development of children with a language disorder, but the pattern of their language is also deviant. Deviancy implies uneven and atypical development. The path to recovery, the eventual emergence of language, may not follow the predictable route. These children may never completely overcome their difficulties and will require a great deal of specialist and professional attention. More than likely, a child with severe language disorder would find the demands of normal school experience overwhelming and require a special environment geared to the needs of language disordered children.

A language disorder might arise in one specific area of the child's language.

Peter, a child of five years, had been described as suffering from dyspraxia, which may be defined as an inability to programme the speech muscles in producing a sequence of acceptable speech sounds. Although he had far less trouble in doing tasks which are not dependent on language and had been assessed by a psychologist as having average non-verbal (or performance) abilities, he had no expressive vocabulary. Peter could not produce a single word and he made himself understood by using signs and gestures, pulling or pointing. Surprisingly, he did demonstrate in his response to instructions, stories and questions, that he understood much of what was said. Peter could not rely on being able to make his speech sounds in the way he intended. Consequently, he never entered any conversations or initiated talk with others.

It might be expected that signs of a child's disability would be present in other aspects of development. Indeed, children with problems in co-ordinating the muscles of the speech organs may have poor fine motor control in hand movements or in using hands and eyes together to do precise tasks, and a generally clumsy way of doing things. In Peter's case the clumsiness was focussed on his tongue and lips. He could not make precise enough movements to suck through a straw or touch a particular point on his lips with his tongue. The fine co-ordination required to produce a rapid sequence of speech sounds was beyond him. Whatever the cause of Peter's speech disability, a great deal of specialised help will be required to overcome or offset the effects of a dyspraxia, with the speech therapist taking a central role in working with the child to help achieve better control of the speech musculature, using a carefully graded sequence of exercises and activities.

The more severe language disorders affect a wide range of language functions, both comprehension and expressive skills. The term *aphasia* has sometimes been used to describe the very rare occasions when a child fails to develop any language at all, or when language is both limited and very different from normal. There is little agreement amongst the experts about the cause of aphasia and it is a term which tends to be applied when all other likely explanations have been ruled out, such as a hearing impairment or mental handicap. It goes without saying that a child who is aphasic, unable to understand or use language appropriately, will be severely hindered in many aspects of learning and development.

Patsy, at four and a half years, had severe problems in understanding spoken language and her parents had to resort to physical means of managing her, such as leading her to the tea-table. She used a few gestures to convey her needs, whilst her own speech was limited to cries, screams and grunts. Not surprisingly, the major difficulties were social ones: Patsy had developed exaggerated emotional responses to change.

Parents spend a lot of time explaining why a child must hurry or wait, what is permitted behaviour and why rules must be followed, and softening the blow of having to go home from a friend's or return a toy, through language. Interestingly, Patsy was aware enough, non-verbally, to understand pictures and diagrams, although she rarely played with dolls or toys. Her parents were able to plan some of the events of the day with Patsy by drawing a timetable of clock-times and picture symbols to denote events, such as getting in the taxi to go to school, shopping with Mother, bedtime, and so on, which was pinned to the kitchen wall. Eventually, Patsy's needs were felt to be so severe that a residential school specialising in helping language-disordered children was recommended. There her gestures were channelled into an established signing system and she soon began to acquire a vocabulary which could be recognised and developed. For Patsy this was felt to be the most appropriate way to help her begin to communicate, in a protective environment where all the staff are expert in using very special techniques and strategies. Patsy may not always require sign language, or such a carefully prepared teaching and living environment. Her parents are delighted that, through giving the child an alternative means of communication, the beginnings of more normal behaviour, relationships, and play, have begun to emerge.

At what point might a special setting be recommended for a child, as opposed to some form of integrated help within a mainstream school? A great deal depends on the individual child and the circumstances and wishes of the family. However, where a child has very severe communication needs requiring intensive help; where the protection and security of small groups is required; where the social and psychological demands of ordinary children are overwhelming; and where there is little meaningful participation in an ordinary class setting, given the resources available; then a special school may be considered.

ENVIRONMENTAL LANGUAGE DIFFICULTIES

One of the issues we shall be addressing at some length in this book is the potential and impetus for learning which most children possess. There are very few children who develop no language at all, providing the conditions for learning are right and the child has suffered no major physical or sensory deficits. That should not be taken to infer that all children develop language at the same rate, or achieve similar degrees of sophistication. There is, however, less agreement on what the basic recipe for growth must include. The main ingredient appears to be early interaction with adults in which the infant is exposed to a consistent speech environment.

It is possible that some environments, both at home and in school, provide much richer opportunities for interactive learning than others. The behaviour of adults involved with children as language novices, together with learning conditions which appear to be optimal, are important areas for research. Knowing what circumstances and strategies appear to be most helpful for the majority of children discovering language informs the approach we take to children with special needs. Inevitably, some children are exposed to less nurturing experiences in the early years and arrive in school less well prepared than others. In the absence of any other problem, such as an underlying intellectual disability, a delay in language might be attributed to limited learning opportunities and inadequate early experience: a kind of 'deprivation'.

There are some rare cases of children whose start in life has been so lacking in the normal patterns of care that it is difficult to see how normal development could take place.

One such case is that of the 'Koluchova' twins, boys of seven years of age discovered in the cellar of a house in Czechoslovakia, in conditions of utter neglect and isolation. Their mother had died soon after giving birth and after a short spell in a children's home the twins went to live with their father and stepmother, who actively rejected them. They were locked up for long periods, slept on the floor on a plastic sheet and were regularly beaten with a rubber hose until they lay flat on the ground unable to move. The boys grew up in almost total isolation. At the time of their discovery they were unable to walk, suffered from malnutrition and had little or no speech. In order to communicate with each other they used gestures. When they saw moving toys, a TV set and traffic for the first time at seven years, they reacted with surprise and horror. During the proceedings for criminal neglect later brought against the parents, neighbours testified that they had often heard inhuman shrieks and howls coming from the cellar, but had not wished to interfere and had no idea of the twins' existence. Subsequently, the twins were fostered in a normal family and their progress monitored. Eventually, the children began to acquire language, made progress in all areas of development, and were able to attend a normal school.

(Koluchova, 1972, 1976)

The unfortunate circumstances of these badly neglected children have helped psychologists to weigh the importance of the early periods of infancy for later development. It has been argued that if children receive little stimulation at the 'critical period' in the first years of life, then irreparable damage occurs. No matter what is done subsequently to help remedy the situation, so the argument runs, if the most sensitive period for language learning is missed, the effects of deprivation will be permanent. To test this hypothesis fully a child would need to be reared in normal conditions but with no opportunity to learn language: a contradiction in terms. In the Koluchova case one would have expected the degree of neglect and maltreatment in themselves would leave life-long scars. However, the fact that the twins grew up to be normally speaking, thinking and loving individuals, following their rescue at seven years, shows that potential for learning survives extreme early deprivation.

A recent review of the handful of known cases where children spent their early years in conditions of severe neglect has been given by Skuse (1984). Common to all these cases is the severe emotional disturbance and grossly delayed development which results from social isolation, but where there are no obvious physical or mental abnormalities in the first place, prognosis is good. When the child is placed in a caring and loving family, recovery is remarkably rapid in all aspects of development, including language. These findings, then, underline the importance of normal social interactions for child development, although the idea of a 'critical period' for learning seems untenable. Perhaps the most important insight from these studies is the tremendous resilience of children.

Thankfully, few teachers will come across children who have suffered such severely depleted environments. However, there are some social circumstances in which children are caught up and which can only be assumed to be harmful. One child we knew was faced with such a rapid succession of caretakers every day, most of whom wanted to keep him asleep and out of the way, that he was never really talked to or played with until he went to school where his poor development was highlighted.

Another child was brought up in a family of hearing-impaired adults who used sign language to communicate. Although normally-hearing, this little girl's only experience of the spoken word came from the television. As a consequence the child had a vivid command of sign, but very delayed speech. In situations of this kind children can be helped by enriching the environment at home or in a nursery. One would expect an environmentally-based problem to resolve in time.

SOCIAL-CLASS DIFFERENCES

It has been a popular belief that children from working-class homes suffer a form of linguistic deprivation which, in turn, leads to relatively poorer achievements in school. This is a complex and controversial subject. A great deal has been written on the factors associated with socio-economic status, particularly intellectual functioning and academic achievement, such as reading. Since social-class differences, whatever these may be, have been said to contribute to important variations in children's language development some of the main issues will be considered briefly here. (For a critical review of many of the influential background studies, see Rutter and Madge, 1976; or Edwards, 1976.)

Perhaps the most influential, but also frequently misinterpreted, of ideas have come from Bernstein (1965). He introduced the notion of an 'elaborated' and a 'restricted' code, or style, of speaking. His interest lies in the way people in different communities use language conceptually, to interact with each other, and to exercise social control. Bernstein wanted to find out how children come to learn socially acceptable behaviour, how they acquire the cultural values and expectations of those around them, and the part played by language therein. His view is that children in different social contexts are exposed to language which leads to different ways of organising experience.

The version of Bernstein's theories which is most well known stems from his early work, where he says that, in some social contexts, children have access only to restricted codes, which limits their powers of expression and thought. A restricted code might be characterised by short, simple sentences, often left unfinished. There might be a narrower range of vocabulary and grammar, with more frequent use of commands, questions and categoric statements ('I'm telling you what to do.'). Restricted speech requires additional information from the context or social setting, in order to be meaningful. There is thus a particular difficulty with abstract concepts. On the other hand, an elaborated code is said to be characterised by complex grammar and vocabulary; use of a wide range of pronouns, prepositions and verb forms; and the flexibility to express complex ideas. An elaborated code can deal with abstract concepts without reference to the immediate context.

Many people took Bernstein's early theories to mean that some children, especially children from the lower working classes, fail to learn in school because they speak a restricted code. The assumption has been made that restricted speech means working-class speech, that this is inferior, and therefore children who use it are badly prepared for the demands of school. Children's *deficits* in language are responsible for educational failure. Bernstein no longer subscribes to the view that social class is directly related to the codes to which a speaker has access. It is also unfair to assume that he was primarily interested in how language causes failure to learn. In his later work (Bernstein, 1973) much greater emphasis was given to the social function of language. Different social groups put different priorities on the way language is used. For example, middle-class mothers may be more likely to explain to a child why they want a change in behaviour, whilst a child in a working-class home may be commanded. The shift in emphasis does not imply that one is better than the other, or that working-class families are unable to use more elaborate codes, when they choose to. The tantalising question remains whether some children's choice of language patterns causes a discontinuity between the culture of the home and of the school.

Despite considerable uncertainty over Bernstein's intended meaning, his work has often been used to support educational policy. What came to be called 'compensatory education' (The Plowden Report, DES, 1967) was based on the view that poverty of language was a major cause of underachievement which the school could offset, and Bernstein's theories (albeit unfairly) were used to support it. The Plowden Report clearly espouses a view that some families have serious shortcomings. These could be compensated for by an expansion of nursery education, direct enrichment of the child's experience in school, and by influencing the parents.

There have been a number of fierce critics of the idea that children from low socio-economic groups are culturally impoverished, hear little well-formed language, cannot convey abstract thoughts, and need a compensatory programme. In a famous paper on the language of black children, Labov (1970) argued that the concept of verbal deprivation is a myth which diverts attention away from the real issues, such as defects in the school system. To put this another way, there are differences, not defects, in the language usage of social class groups. Labov shows in some detail that the language of Negro children is just as logically complex as any other. *Schools* fail by presenting an alien social situation to some children, in which they do not learn and are not expected to do so. It is sometimes believed that Labov and Bernstein are bitterly opposed to each other, but that is not strictly true.

In Britain, Tough (1976) has more recently put forward the view that there are social-class differences in the uses to which language is put. The disadvantaged children in her study rarely used language for logical reasoning, sequencing events, making comparisons, predicting events or recalling the past, reflecting on problems and other people's feelings, and in imaginative play. In Tough's view, such children hear language used in more limited ways at home: to control ('Sit still') and to label ('That's a fire engine'); but less often in reflection or explanation. Addressing herself largely to teachers, Tough designed a scheme for appraising and developing more complex language usage in working-class children.

Despite its wide acceptance, the belief in linguistic deprivation associated with social disadvantage is based on very flimsy evidence. Few researchers have actually bothered to record the conversations which are held in working-class homes to uphold the notion that parents do not talk to their children or make complex use of language. In fact, those few studies where the home context has been investigated show few differences in the amount of mother-child talk, length of conversations, or the frequency and nature of questions. Both middle- and working-class families can be observed using complex language of an explicit kind, in giving explanations and information, and in developing concepts. There are, however, great individual differences between children as well as between children's behaviour in different settings.

One of the most important findings of the research by Tizard and Hughes (1984) relates to the gulf between working-class children's interactions with their mothers at home and with their teachers in school. Radio-microphone recordings were made in the family and in nursery school, to give a picture of the separate language environments. In all family contexts, irrespective of social class, a richness of talk, interaction and intellectual challenge is depicted, an endless 'asking and answering' of questions (op. cit, page 73). The picture changes markedly for all children in nursery school. Interactions between adult and child are fewer and briefer in the nursery, whilst the style of conversation shifts towards greater use of commands and questions. Significantly, it is the working-class children who suffer most in nursery: teachers make fewer demands on them, whilst they make fewer approaches to staff. A large discrepancy appears between the quality and amount of language interaction experienced at home and in school by the working-class children.

It is essential that teachers know something of the 'verbal deprivation' arguments that have been propounded. The common-sense view of this research is that all children are different, most family settings provide rich sources of learning, but some school contexts fail to complement the vividness of many homes. This is, of course, in stark contrast to what many teachers believe happens. Working-class homes are not often claimed to be more powerful learning environments than school. Two major things can be learned from this: not to make sweeping generalisations about class or 'disadvantage'; and always to think out how the school setting can respond more effectively to a child's needs, rather than risking a misjudgement about a child's capabilities on the basis of social expectations. In the book by Edwards (1979) on the relationship between social class and language development, an important warning is sounded for teachers:

> In every case, the aim must be to assist the child in developing his fullest potential. Anything which proves an obstacle in this process should be carefully examined to ascertain whether it is a substantial difficulty or whether it is a product of social attitude. As we have seen, a child's language, which to many teachers can appear to represent the former category is, in most instances, a manifestation of the latter.
>
> (op. cit. page 139)

THE PROBLEM WITH CATEGORIES

Earlier in this chapter we gave some basic definitions of language handicaps and illustrated these with descriptions of individual children. However, we would not wish teachers to believe that children fit neatly into pigeonholes, and this is particularly true of the ramifications of a stereotype such as 'socially disadvantaged'. Categories are sometimes useful ways of summarising and contrasting complex individual differences. In the context of language development it is important to know what these typologies mean, whilst also appreciating that there are usually considerable overlaps between divisions. A child's language behaviour at one moment in time has a unique and complex relationship with background experience, abilities and development, together with influences in the present context in which communication takes place. It is also true that any language difficulty, even a very mild problem in articulating speech sounds, spills over into other areas of development such as social confidence, and cannot be considered in isolation.

There is a danger, too, that the nomenclature we use colours our expectations and views of the child. If we group children together under some medical-sounding label we might expect them to share a known underlying cause, to behave in the same way and produce identical symptoms, and to respond to the same course of treatment. The medical model is an inappropriate way of looking at the field of language difficulties, because, in the majority of children, we do not know the underlying aetiology, and even if we did, the patterns of language displayed by individuals would show no straightforward correspondence with the cause. Children must be approached as unique personalities. The particular circumstances of a child's home; the school setting; style of learning; the way the child relates to others; response to experience; what is learned quickly or poorly; and the individual profile of achievement in different skill areas – all these produce a spectrum of features unique to the child.

Some children become victims of their handicap because a label is attached to them with self-fulfilling prophecies. For example, if it is generally believed that a profound hearing loss precludes children from developing normal speech, achieving highly in academic subjects, and participating in normal social situations, then teacher-expectations will be lowered, fewer demands will be made, and less challenges offered. This will apply to all children who suffer under the label, no matter how competent or determined they are to succeed.

The problem with categories, too, is that teachers are encouraged to attribute every difficulty which arises to the child's disability. We assume that the learning problems experienced by the child, lie *within* the child, because of the handicap. There is a growing awareness that it is not just children who have special needs: teachers also have special needs. Teachers, classroom practice and schools themselves, vary enormously in their effectiveness. Knowing that leaves the way forward to changing the way adults behave, the strategies teachers adopt, and the conditions for learning. In other words, we do not accept that because children are language-disordered or socially disadvantaged they will therefore fail to learn; instead, we identify strategies and situations through which children are helped to learn more effectively.

Labels and categories are thus no more than a starting point in our thinking about individuals. They do not explain a child, or help a teacher to do a more effective job. What is important is that teachers know something about the parameters by which a child's particular difficulties can be defined. How can we observe and describe the individual's linguistic behaviour? What kind of theoretical framework will help us to analyse and understand the feature of a child's language system, and plan appropriate teaching intervention? In the following chapter we shall be addressing these questions in some detail. We shall be looking at descriptive continua such as the child's intelligibility, comprehension of meaning and mastery of the structure of language. These dimensions at least allow us to say something of the individual, the child's capabilities as well as limitations, without falling into the pitfalls associated with labels and categories.

SPECIAL NEEDS AND RECENT LEGISLATION

At the time of writing, the Warnock Report (DES, 1978) has become a familiar discussion piece to teachers, whilst local authorities are still working through their legal responsibilities to children with 'special needs' in the wake of the 1981 Education Act. The report of the Warnock Committee, and the legislation which stemmed from its findings, have important implications for all children with learning difficulties, not least of all those with a significant language handicap. It is not the intention to cover the details of the Warnock inquiry or the recent legislation in any depth here. However, the general principles which underlie the new Act reflect a changed emphasis in our view of special needs. A great deal of what we have to say in this book about language difficulties shares this new emphasis, particularly with regard to the assessment and monitoring of children, the issue of integration, and the involvement of parents.

Prior to the 1981 Education Act, special education had always been defined in terms of a child's disability. Categories such as ESN(S) were used to label children and then determine the kind of educational provision which was required. This led to a view of special education as being synonymous with special schools, units or classes. The numbers of children involved might be around two per cent of the total school population. The Warnock committee recommended a much broader view of special education. To take just two of the goals which teachers usually adopt in school, increasing a child's understanding of the world and achieving independence, for example – a special educational need is defined by whatever obstacles the child has to face in working toward these goals. Special educational help can also be defined in terms of whatever extra assistance is required, however and wherever this is provided, in order to overcome a learning difficulty. The importance of this view of special education is that it moves the focus of attention away from categories of handicap and the child's disability, towards the environment in which the child must learn.

Under the 1981 Act, professionals are no longer to use categories of handicap in determining a child's special needs, and the practice of fitting children up with labels such as 'dyslexic', 'dyspraxic' or 'ESN(M)' is discouraged. Educational needs are to be thought of in terms of a *continuum*. At one end of the scale there are children whose learning difficulties are easily overcome; at the other end a child may be severely hindered in achievement. In terms of language difficulties there are many children whose immaturity of speech sounds persists, but who are not really affected in their learning. At the far end of the scale, however, a central problem of using and processing language will significantly affect the child's overall development. To reiterate, then, what the teacher requires professionally, in order to identify and describe a child's language difficulty, is a working knowledge of the continua of linguistic skills important in development.

Whatever the exact figures involved, the Warnock view implies that many more children may have special needs at some point in their school careers than was hitherto recognised. In fact the Warnock Report suggested that one in five children may have special needs, a figure based partly on large-scale studies of whole populations of children, such as the Isle of Wight Survey (Rutter, Tizard, and Whitmore, 1970). To meet these needs special education has to become a wider and more flexible process, capable of adjusting to the individual. Obviously, the Warnock view embraces many children already within ordinary schools. It advocates that we should no longer differentiate between those children who attend special schools and those who do not. However we help a child, whether through additional speech therapy or teaching help, withdrawal to special classes, or special school referral, can be seen as part of a continuum of response to specific children's needs.

ENGLISH AS A SECOND LANGUAGE

The Warnock Report and the legislation which stemmed from it made some important points about the special needs of children with English as a second language. Many teachers have had the experience of a child arriving in school with very little English, whose family's mother tongue may have been Chinese, Punjabi, Italian, or so on. In an inner London primary school in which one of the authors worked, the head teacher prided himself on the fact that 23 different languages were represented amongst just over 100 children. Obviously, that would be an immediate problem in a school where the language of instruction and of social contact is English. Teachers have a demanding job in such a situation and in many local authorities there are language support teams staffed by skilled people, who have developed strategies to help children acquire English and therefore participate in the learning experience.

The Swann Report (DES, 1985) has recently explored the ways in which local education authorities and individual schools and teachers should respond to the needs of a multi-racial society. In enlightened authorities respect is paid to the cultural traditions associated with ethnic minority groups, so that they do not lose their distinctive features. There is no reason why the contrasting life-styles, social customs, folklore, religious beliefs and artistic heritage of different cultural groups should not enrich the classroom experience for all children. The Swann Report guards against 'tokenism': paying lip-service to different ethnic groups by teaching about them in the classroom, without really changing underlying attitudes or preparing children for life in a pluralist society.

In some areas children are taught initially in their mother tongues, whilst others withdraw children to teach English in separate classes. There is usually a varied response to such practices, with some teachers feeling that both isolate children. In a few people's minds, when children are exposed to more than one language at home and in school, they are felt to be linguistically disadvantaged. The Swann Report suggests that the learning of English should be the genuine concern of all teachers, with the practice of withdrawing children to teach English as a second language abandoned. Using the child's mother tongue as a medium of instruction and fostering a child's fluency in the home language are both seen positively.

Not surprisingly, all these issues are very contentious ones, with few straightforward solutions. In fact the majority of children in the world are brought up in multi-lingual settings. There is very little evidence that children will be confused, slower, or limited by having to learn more than one language at once. In the ordinary course of events children naturally learn whatever languages are used around them. What is true, however, is that educational systems are dominated by high status languages in the sense that those who use them are held in high regard. It is a peculiar paradox that we congratulate a British child who manages to learn enough French in school to be able to converse confidently on holidays, whilst at the same time fail to acknowledge the achievements of a seven-year old immigrant child with three or four low status languages at its fingertips. The Swann Report suggests, for example, that in schools where there are a large number of speakers of a particular community language, then this could form part of the modern languages on offer in the school concerned.

When the situation arises where a non-English speaking child arrives in school, it should be recognised that the child may have less difficulty in learning than the teacher has in teaching. Such children may quickly develop a superficial fluency in English which later prompts an interpretion of a learning disability when the child fails to grasp some more complex or abstract concept. It has been said that it takes at least five years for a balanced bilingual ability to emerge (Cummins, 1984). Problems can arise for children who grow up with a superficial command of a new language, particularly if immigrant parents are advised to use the host language at home and the first language is forgotten.

To reiterate: issues in second language learning are complex and compounded by social and cultural status. The 1981 Education Act says that a child should not be thought to have special needs solely because the language spoken at home is different from that used in school. The Warnock view is that a child's educational difficulties should be assessed with due reference to cultural background, the demands of living in a new social setting and possible material disadvantages or confusions in identity. Sensitive attention should be paid to the testing of children in a second language, giving parents information in an understandable form and access to a professional who speaks their language. The intention of the new legislation is not to deny immigrant groups the protection or benefits of the special needs procedures, nor to subject them to the law unnecessarily. The essential issue is that English as a second language does not, of itself, create learning difficulties for the child. This is, therefore, one group of children we shall not be discussing further in the context of speech and language difficulties in school.

INTEGRATION

Integration is not an end in itself. The aims of education, what we hope our teaching is working towards, remain the same for all children, whatever their needs. Integration is a process and not a goal. As such it encompasses a wide variety of practices. A child with special needs in speech and language who participates entirely without extra help in a normal class, perhaps visited weekly by a speech therapist, might be described as 'integrated'. For another child 'integration' may mean that a special language class is attended in the morning at an ordinary school with the child entering mainstream groups in the afternoon. At the far extreme a child who attends a special school because of severe communication needs, may visit a nearby comprehensive school with a teacher for an 'integrated' period of games or metalwork. Integration should be judged on how much *real* sharing of learning experiences, play, mealtimes and social activities takes place. In the end, as we have said, it is the child's educational gains which are paramount. If the child is not learning through an integrated experience, it is a pointless exercise.

It is sometimes believed that children who are integrated into ordinary schools are those who would otherwise be in special classes or schools. The thinking behind the 1981 Education Act tries to remove this assumption. The wider concept of special needs proposes that many children, some of them unrecognised, have learning difficulties requiring additional help. To respond individually to each child's needs requires flexible strategies, arrangements geared to the child and the situation. Integration is not, then, an either/or question. It is one kind of teaching process available for helping children with varying degrees of learning difficulty within the ordinary school.

Under the 1981 Education Act, local authorities have a general duty to help as many children as possible with special needs in mainstream schools. In principle, children cannot be excluded because of the nature or severity of their disability. However, the 1981 Act is not a charter for closing special schools down and returning every child to mainstream. Several major conditions must be satisfied for integration to take place. Education in the mainstream must be compatible with the child receiving the special help required. Integration must represent an 'efficient use of resources' and not interfere with the education of the ordinary majority of children. The new legislation, *per se*, is unlikely to produce new initiatives for integration, to change attitudes or existing policy. What it does do, is to give parents the right to ask for their child to have some integrated experience with ordinary children. More importantly, it recognises the wider responsibilities of ordinary schools and teachers towards children with learning difficulties, many of whom go undetected and without help.

The recent thinking about special needs fits together very well with the approach we have adopted towards children who experience communication problems. To the question 'Where should children with language difficulties be helped?', we would answer that a normal speech environment is a good starting point. Most children learn more quickly and effectively in the company of children who make appropriate linguistic demands and at the right interest level, upon each other. There are very few children whose communication handicaps are so severe that they cannot take a meaningful part, for some of the day, in a normal school situation. The majority of children addressed in this book are to be found in normal schools. To the question 'Whose problem is a language handicap?' we would answer that a team approach is warranted with specialists, teachers, and parents sharing their own particular insights to help plan for the child.

WORKING TOGETHER

At several points in this book we shall be arguing that speech and language problems cannot be treated directly or in isolation, and we should focus our energies on the conditions which help the child to learn most effectively. That may stand in stark contrast to how some professionals are thought to operate. Speech therapists, for example, have often been cast in the role of clinicians who 'treat' patients at a clinic. Some children and their caregivers, indeed, view such visits as they might a trip to the dentist, for an inspection and any necessary repair work. In some school situations, speech therapy sessions are organised on the same basis as physiotherapy might be, with the child going out of the class for a ten minute session. This is, in fact, a practice common to all kinds of 'remedial' work, even to the extent of some children attending reading clinics.

Whilst there may be a perfectly good argument for using specialist resources in this way to help individual children, there is another way of looking at the issue. If, as we have argued, language is an integral part of everything that children do in the classroom, why remove children from the learning context in order to try and improve their skills? It is often noted that what the child learns in a remedial group or speech therapy session does not generalise to the classroom situation. When that happens it makes clear sense to move towards a much closer working relationship between professionals. Many speech therapists now recognise the important contributions that they can make in organising and devising a language programme with the teacher or parent, in a natural and spontaneous language learning context.

This line of argument we extend to all professionals involved with children experiencing speech and language difficulties. In one area a university department of linguistics is directly involved in the assessment of children referred to it through the speech therapy service and in suggesting intervention strategies. Linguists have a particularly taxing job of translating academic theory into the kind of practice which is accessible to non-specialists who care for the child from day to day, both at home and in school. So too, medical officers and educational psychologists have a responsibility to share information amongst one another and with the most significant adults in the child's life: parents and teachers. Professionals must be careful not to usurp the role of parents or teachers. If we believe in the interactionist view of language-learning, then the proper contribution of the 'experts' is towards helping children in their social and school contexts. We shall have more to say about professional roles and the stages at which different agencies may become involved with a child who gives rise to concern, in chapter 3.

THE IMPORTANCE OF PARENTS

The three most frequent sources of complaint by parents of children with special needs are: they are given inadequate information, they are offered unrealistic advice, and what they as parents have to say is ignored (Tumin, 1978). Many parents feel dissatisfied with the advice given by 'experts', whilst they also lose confidence in their own abilities to help their child. It is not uncommon for different experts to give conflicting views and suggestions – which produces a great deal of anxiety, confusion and misinterpretation.

Perhaps the most far-reaching implications of the 1981 Education Act concern the more central role which parents should play in assessment, decision-making, planning and teaching. As in many instances where children have special needs, it is often the parents who register the first concern about a child's language development. Parents should have access to advice and support services, should be kept fully informed, and should be dealt with honestly and openly. The precise implications of the recent legislation for teachers in relation to parents are set out in chapter 3. But, at this point, it is important to stress that parents are usually intimately conversant with their own child's personality and learning style and are often well motivated to help themselves, given positive advice.

One astounding fact about normal language development is that by the age at which children are often admitted to nursery classes, around three years of age, most children have a sophisticated grasp of the major elements of the language system and have already begun to think logically and enquiringly about the environment. These active efforts to make sense of a complex world begin, by and large, in the context of the home. No-one can deny the importance of these early years in terms of the child's first explorations, social relationships and intellectual growth. Where a child is experiencing special developmental difficulties, we advocate, as others have done (Chazan et al., 1980), early advice and help. Parents continue to play the key role and should be able to work in partnership with any supplementary support from, say, a speech therapist, pre-school counsellor or nursery group.

We have already made reference to the important work by Tizard and Hughes (1984) which questions the myth of verbal deprivation in working-class families. Equally disturbing, to these authors, is the myth that professionals are better at fostering children's development than parents. The nursery teachers in this study provided children with much less frequent and intense interaction than did the parents, with a greater emphasis on informal play. Children often failed to respond to the questioning approach of the teachers, and, because staff did not know the children as closely as their mothers, conversations were less likely to be as sustained or as free-ranging.

To summarise: both working- and middle-class homes provided a rich learning experience for the child, different in kind and more intense than the nursery class. It is worth remembering, then, that a good nursery should supplement and not supplant the child's experience at home.

2

The normal developmental process

Allgone drink
Panda eated it dinner
What she can sit in?
Pussy bringed in some mouses

These utterances are recognisably those of ordinary young children learning language. In the early stages children miss out words, use the wrong word endings, change the order of words around, and often put sentences together quite differently from the way adults do. These language patterns are anticipated by adults, who shape their own responses accordingly to help the language novice; for example, by checking and expanding on what the child intended to say and presenting a better sentence model:

Child: Panda eated it dinner.
Adult: Yes, Panda's eaten all his dinner.

What makes these sentences so different from the example given at the beginning of chapter 1? (Him no got none Peter.) In the earlier extract what the child says has such an unusual organisation that an uneasy gap opens between the child and the listener. We can hazard a guess that this child often experiences a breakdown in his talk with others. Adults intuitively know, however, how to respond to the typically immature language of ordinary children, exemplified above. In this chapter we shall be looking primarily at what we know of the normal process of language acquisition. Perhaps the most engaging research question of all is how children move from being language novice to language expert in such a short space of time. However, we can learn a great deal about how to help children with special needs in speech and language, by observing the behaviour and experiences of ordinary children.

It would be wrong to think that the process of language development only begins when children use their first words. Important learning takes place before children start to talk in the early games mothers share with their children, such as 'Peek-a-boo', when turn-taking (first you, then me) is experienced. It is also clear from everyday observation that children do not learn simply by *imitating* the speech of adults. Few adults use phrases such as 'We haved some gingerbread mens', or 'my bestest picture'. An important insight can be drawn from these early 'mistakes' of children. Right from the outset children can be observed extracting rules from what they hear in language and then applying these rules to what they have to say for themselves, so that in the early stages children's language shows these characteristic differences from the adult patterns.

Recently, researchers have begun to look at the wider context in which children acquire language. It is not enough to describe children's vocabulary or grammar, without looking at what children are trying to do with language, and whether they succeed. The emphasis has shifted to language as communication. By thinking about children interacting with their adult caretakers, busily engaged in *using* language together, we begin to glimpse the purposeful nature of the whole process. At the end of this chapter, when we summarise what seem to be the most facilitating factors in normal children developing language, our focus is very largely on the environment and the behaviour of adults, rather than the child. It has taken some time for researchers to realise that language blossoms within a very special growing medium, supplied quite unconsciously by the child's caregivers.

It goes without saying that the patterns of development we can observe in healthy young children as they grow, are both vividly complex and intricately interwoven. Faced with a minutiae of observations, psychologists always respond by constructing a model. A model is a means of simplifying detail in order to understand the overall processes at work. In this chapter we shall be looking at models which help us to understand how, in the ordinary course of events, the central aspects of normal language development unfold. It is important to start with the normal developmental process for several reasons. Firstly, having a clear framework of language acquisition and behaviour for the ordinary child provides us with important yardsticks when we come to consider the child who is suspected to be atypical. Having said that, the observer of so-called 'normal' children is usually surprised at the infinite variety found. However, the essence of a theoretical model is that it gives some clear cut, if hypothetical, bench-marks.

The second major reason for beginning with normal developmental processes is that, for the teacher, knowing the skills children usually acquire stage-by-stage provides important guidelines for both assessment and teaching. When we come to consider ways of identifying and appraising the special language needs of a particular child, the teacher's best insights will not come via formal tests, language batteries, or vocabulary lists, but from a clear understanding of what is appropriate behaviour for a child of a certain age. Just as importantly, knowing *how* children normally progress through a sequence of skills, and the experiences which enable them to do so, is the teacher's 'highway code'. The teacher who grasps this will be able to plan natural learning steps for the child, to formulate realistic and appropriate teaching objectives, and to evaluate the effectiveness of the teaching/learning experience.

A word of caution is necessary. If we have selected or lifted some aspects of language development out of their social contexts, this is simply to make them accessible. However, this is one example of human behaviour where the sum is always greater than its parts. It should be borne in mind that every level of the child's language behaviour is intimately related to social, emotional and intellectual factors, as well as to important variables outside of the child, in particular the social environment in which children find themselves and in which language is used.

ASPECTS OF LANGUAGE

It is important to be clear about what we are going to include in our model of language development. Some linguists feel that there are only certain kinds of communication which can properly be called 'language'. Auditory–vocal communication involving hearing and speech is obviously the primary medium of language. Some of the properties of speech are also shared by language represented visually in written form or in sign. The most important property is the creative potential of these forms of language: their *productivity*. Words and word-combinations in speech, books and sign language are continually being invented and have an infinite potential of meaningful variations, depending on how the user puts them together. Furthermore, it is possible to distinguish between two levels of language: meaningless segments such as letters and sounds; and the larger units when the basic elements are sequenced in a particular way to express meaning. These defining properties of language, creativity and duality of structure, exclude some gestures or body language from being 'linguistic' in the true sense of the word. For example, smiling, turning away or raising the eyebrows, are forms of communication which are non-linguistic. However, some gestures and body signals do constitute part of a linguistic system, as in the case of British Sign Language. In BSL a raised backward hand movement to indicate past tense can be used in relation with other signs to produce novel messages.

The essence of a language, then, is that a knowledge of it enables the user to produce an infinite number of new sentences which may

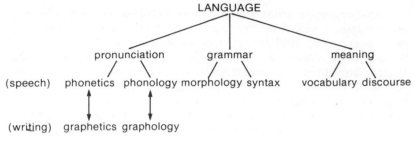

Figure 2.1 Model of language structure (adapted from Crystal, 1976)

never have been used before, but which can still be understood by anyone else familiar with the same language. Very often, a distinction is drawn between the two processes of producing and receiving language forms. The reception or comprehension of speech includes the hearing and discrimination of sounds. Children need to be able to focus attention on the sounds they hear, as a first step towards interpreting their meaning. The development of receptive language is traditionally felt to precede expressive skill, so that many children are able to understand more complex sentence patterns than the language they themselves can produce. A more current view is that receptive and expressive language may develop interactively, with productive language ahead of receptive for some of the time. For example, from the age of about three years, children may say words they do not understand, or use intonation patterns without being fully aware of all their meanings. Expressive language, too, depends on a spectrum of factors for development, including sensory, intellectual, motor and social aspects. It is perfectly possible for children who are unable to talk to have a normal understanding of language. In this sense, language refers to the child's access to inner verbal concepts as a mode of thinking about, categorising and shaping experience. The classic book by Furth (1966) attempted to show that some deaf children with poor speech are not devoid of language and can perform complex intellectual tasks requiring sophisticated inner concepts.

A model of the main branches of the field of linguistics is given in figure 2.1, taken from Crystal (1976). This provides a very clear summary of the important features of language, how they are interrelated and how they may be studied. This model is not concerned with language in use, simply separate levels of the structure of language. We shall have much more to say about language in use – the ways in which the structure of language varies in relation to the social context – later on in this chapter.

The left-hand side of this diagram, under the heading 'pronunciation', is concerned with the *sounds* of a language. The study of the range of sounds which human beings are able to produce with the vocal apparatus at their disposal is called 'phonetics'. Whilst a very wide range of sounds can be produced, only a small set of sounds is used in any particular language to express meanings. Sounds are organised into a system of contrasts and words are distinguished from each other by the substitution of one type of sound for another. As an example, 'him' is discriminated from 'hid' by the contrast between 'm' and 'd' at the end of the words. In the English language there are only a limited number of these contrastive units. The 'phonology' of the sound system of English refers to the 40 or so distinctive sound units which we use in pronouncing words, and which are known as phonemes.

Still on this left-hand side of the tree diagram, we can study the way in which a language's spelling and punctuation system is constructed. Just as the sounds of a language can be described, a corresponding approach can be made to its written features. The wider range of human mark-making is called 'graphetics', whereas analysis of the particular written patterns of a specific language has been called 'graphology' (Crystal, 1976, page 27). In the same way as each language has a distinctive phonological system, so too, each language has its own range of graphemes: the special units of writing which are used to set the language down on paper.

Learning to read has sometimes been described in terms of establishing correspondences between the grapheme–phoneme features of the language. This 'phonic' approach stresses the links which exist in *regular* words between the printed symbols of the alphabet and the sounds of speech. The child's attention can be drawn to the distinctive letter sounds, so that initial attempts at reading become a process of learning the rules for decoding print into sound. We shall be returning to this issue again in chapter 3 when we discuss reading and writing difficulties in relation to underlying language skills. It is sufficient to note at this point that the importance of phonemic or phonological aspects of learning to read is under dispute, largely because much of the vocabulary the child meets in reading is irregular and a set of phonic strategies, however well mastered, will only get the child so far in reading for meaning.

In relation to the language model in figure 2.1, grapheme–phoneme aspects of language and reading occupy a peripheral position. The central part of the diagram, significantly, is taken up by grammar. Grammar can be looked at in two respects. Firstly, the way in which word structures change (sleep, sleeping, slept, asleep) is described as 'morphology'. The second, and perhaps more crucial aspect, is the study of syntax. Syntax accounts for the way in which words are fitted together in phrase, clause and sentence patterns, to form an organised and meaningful sequence. Grammar takes the central role because it is the child's internal knowledge and control of the rules and organising principles of language which enable sounds to be related to meaning. Without the structure of grammar language would remain a random collocation of sounds and ideas. There are good reasons to believe that the child's growing understanding of the grammatical patterns of language is just as important for the skill of reading, as knowing about sounds.

The right-hand side of the tree diagram is occupied by meaning. This area of language study is perhaps the most complicated, if only because we cannot observe meaning – it has to be inferred. Linguists have tried to analyse meaning by establishing what it is that individual words convey, how meaning is distributed amongst the different parts of a sentence, and how it arises from the interaction of its separate elements. These are fairly static approaches to meaning, or 'semantics' as it is sometimes called, akin to looking up a word in a dictionary or translating a French expression into its English equivalent. When we come to consider how meaning arises in children's development of language, we cannot approach the problem in isolation. To discover how meaning develops, attention must be paid to the social context in which language is used, how children interact with their caretakers, and the strategies which are adopted by which meaning is communicated to another.

THE DEVELOPMENT OF SOUNDS

Children move through a series of stages as they acquire the distinctive sound contrasts of English. In the first stage, the baby's sounds are usually crying, cooing, laughing, gurgling and a range of vocalisations which register hunger, discomfort or pleasure. This is often felt to be a practice phase, prior to the production of speech sounds proper, when the baby develops fine control of tongue, lips and speech muscles. It has been noticed that the early vocalisations of hearing-impaired babies up to the age of about six months are similar to those of normally-hearing children. This suggests that the early practice phase does not depend on children being able to hear the speech of those around them. Babies from different language backgrounds also show little influence of the home language and produce the same kind of vocalisations at this stage.

The task that lies ahead of the child is to work out how to produce sounds and then to find out which sounds are used by the speakers around them. So, fairly quickly, the child *is* influenced by the speech sounds heard and vocalisation becomes much more purposeful and speechlike, with sounds like consonants, vowels, and their combination and repetition, appearing. This is usually referred to as the 'babble' stage. Sounds not used in the speech environment drop out of the child's babble. Features such as rhythm, tone of voice and intonation, take on the characteristics of the specific language used around the child. In the case of the hearing-impaired child, by the end of the first year of infancy a deaf child's vocalisations would be recognisably fewer, flatter and less rhythmical, with much less variation in tone than those of the hearing child.

From about nine months onwards infants begin to use sounds consistently which can be interpreted as first words. Delighted parents may recognise attempts at 'Mama' or 'Dada' on the basis of rhythm and intonation. The child may use such a word to express a whole host of meanings, questions and needs. For example, one child used 'bo-bo' to refer to her feeding bottle and with a range of gestures, pointing and intonation, 'bo-bo' could mean 'I need a drink', together with 'my bottle is lost', as well as 'this is too hot'. At this stage children recognise different meanings conveyed in the tone or rise and fall of an adult's voice, and use these features themselves. The work of Halliday (1975) referred to in the first chapter shows that, even before recognisable words are used, infants are capable of expressing a wide variety of intentions, demands and meanings through sounds, rhythms and intonation patterns.

Once a child has begun to use words, the sound contrasts which signify different meanings begin to be built up step-by-step. During the earlier practice and babble stages, a wide range of sounds may have been used, but it is only at about 12 months of age that sound contrasts begin to be organised meaningfully. In other words the infant learns the sound distinctions which account for the differences between words such as 'tap', 'top', 'hop', 'mop', 'map', 'gap', and so on. Accounts of the sequence of development of speech sounds are given in Dale (1976) and Ingram (1976). The process is long and not fully understood. Whilst children do vary in the order in which they begin to use individual sounds, there are some general tendencies which can be described.

Most children control consonant sounds such as 'b', 'm', 'p' or 'w', produced at the front of the mouth, before back consonants such as 'k' or 'g'. So too, children often simplify the pronunciation of words with many sounds, such as 'cho-cho' for 'chocolate'. In the early stages almost all children reduce the sounds in clusters of consonants that begin words to a single consonant. So 'drink' becomes 'dink', 'spoon' becomes 'poon' and 'smartie', 'martie'. Between the ages of two and three years children begin to hear contrasts in speech sounds although they might be unable to produce some distinctions. A daughter of one of the authors resisted teasing about the 'sh'/'f' confusions in her own speech, although she clearly *heard* the contrast:

Adult: Here's a frog, see.
Child: And another shog.
Adult: Put that shog in the bucket.
Child: It's not a shog, it's a *shog*.

It is universal, then, for children to pronounce words with some sounds missing, others changed, and yet others substituted. The child is busy working out the systematic rules for pronouncing words. One youngster went through a phase of substituting 't' for 'k' sounds which resulted in 'tornbeef' for 'cornbeef', 'toffee' for 'coffee' and 'toolbox' instead of 'coolbox'. Eventually, and not often beyond five years of age, children bring their own pronunciation rules into line with those of adults. Occasionally, a child will continue to have difficulties with certain sounds in some words, such as the complex sequence of sounds in 'toothbrush', 'scratch', 'probably', or 'umbrella'. A word like 'twelfth' or 'rhinoceros' may not be mastered until nine or ten years.

Knowing the different stages which children pass through in their development of phonological skills is important for two reasons. Firstly, it enables a judgement to be made on the relative maturity of one child's sound system compared with the norm. Secondly, a framework of reference based on what normal children do tempers intuitive judgements about what is typical or atypical. For example, it is usual for children to babble sounds in the pre-word stage which disappear as the child begins to learn how to use speech sounds more systematically. This is an observation often made about hearing-impaired children, that they appear to 'stop talking'. But it can also be observed in normally-hearing children that fluency falters as the babbling stage of practising a range of sounds moves into the organisation of more meaningful speech. One child who produced a perfect 'turtle' at 15 months to refer to a toy in his bath, later began to say 'kurka' in keeping with the way he said other words at this time (de Villiers and de Villiers, 1979).

THE DEVELOPMENT OF GRAMMAR

In the same way that the sequence of events in acquiring sounds can be charted, so too there is a general pattern in the stages children go through in mastering the grammar of their language. Here too it should be borne in mind that there can be tremendous differences between children, as well as variations *within* the individual, in the rate at which different skills are acquired. What seems to hold true is that all normal children pass through similar stages of language growth towards the adult language in a predictable sequence. Some children do this more or less quickly than others and there may be many overlaps between stages. In recent years linguists have been particularly interested in highlighting the features associated with the separate stages of grammatical development (see, for example, Crystal, Fletcher, and Garman, 1976).

Stage 1

The first words usually appear, as we have already said, by 9 to 12 months. It is not uncommon for a child of eight months to be using words, whilst some 18-month-old infants have yet to attempt a recognisable word. At this fairly primitive linguistic stage, from 9 to 18 months, the child's sentences are typically single element, such as 'more', 'biccy', 'teddy', 'gone', 'hot', and 'bye-bye'. The things that children talk about first tend to be objects around them in the here and now. Nelson (1973) studied the first ten words used by a group of 18 children, and the categories most frequently referred to were animals, food and toys. By the time these children had vocabularies of 50 words, at approximately two years, words were used for vehicles (boat, car), clothing (shoe, sock), body parts (nose, ear), and people (mama, baby).

In the first stage children may express negation by shaking the head, frowning or using the word 'no'. A question word such as 'what?' or 'where?' might be used, together with an appropriate gesture, facial expression, or intonation pattern. Not a great deal can be said about the grammar of these early utterances. It is tempting, in view of the range of meanings expressed, to credit the child with a greater understanding of grammar than is warranted. For example, a child may use the word 'light' with a rising intonation which could mean 'Can you put the light on/off?', 'Is that object hanging from the ceiling a light?', or 'I want to go to sleep'. One rule of thumb in making a purely grammatical assessment of a child is to avoid interpreting what the child means. However, if we accept that the most important function of language is to communicate, then we cannot disregard the child's intention in using language, however limited the grammar.

Stage II

By the time a child has acquired around 50 words, that is between the age of about 18 and 24 months, single utterances begin to be combined to make sentence patterns with two elements of structure. Typical of this second stage are sentences such as 'There shoe', 'Dolly bed', 'Daddy read', 'Coat off', 'Teddy sleep.' Children may apply a well-used word such as 'more', 'all-gone' or 'naughty' to a range of others: 'naughty doggy', 'naughty baby', 'not naughty'. A child may use the same two elements to express different meanings. 'Mummy car' could be used in one context to mean 'Mummy's gone to work in the car', whilst in another context, the child means 'Help me into the car.'

The child at this stage will have learnt some negative forms, such as placing 'no' or 'not' in front of an utterance – 'no juice', 'not fall', 'nomore biccy'. Similarly, the main question words used are 'where' or 'what' attached to the beginning of a response. For example, a child may ask 'Where Mummy?' or 'What that?' with a rising intonation. More than likely, children will also ask about things and make requests by non-verbal gestures, such as pointing or looking alternatively at the object and then at the listener. Open-handed reaching and grasping gestures, together with tugging at the clothes and hands of an adult, can be observed in many pre-school children.

Stage III

At the third stage of grammatical development, between approxi-mately 24 and 30 months, children begin to use sentences containing three main elements. Function words like prepositions (in, to, of), pronouns (I, he, they), and determiners (the, my, that), enable the child to relate words and express more elaborate meanings. Word endings like plural noun forms or the past tense of verbs are added. From what children hear used around them, hypotheses are formed, for example, that more than one object can be expressed by adding an 's' at the end of the word: 'boy – boys', 'apple – apples'. The idea that children learn language by constructing such rules for themselves, rather than by imitating adults, comes from the systematic errors made at this stage: 'mouses', 'breads', 'tooths'. Hypotheses are tested out against the reactions of others to what the child says and whether the child succeeds in putting the intended meaning across. Some examples of sentences at this stage are 'Pussy wants milk', 'Give teddy Dada', 'My dolly crying.'

It is around this third stage that children begin to acquire the different verb auxiliaries and suffixes which mark tense. Knowing how to refer to past or future events is a big step forward since children are then released from the 'here and now' and cannot only talk about things which have happened, but can also plan what they are going to do next. This could be seen as a major influence on 'disembedded' or abstract thinking: talking about things which are not immediately present and which have to be imagined. In English, the different past tense suffixes may take some time to sort out. Children might pick up a past tense form like 'broke', 'ran', 'brought' or 'ate', before really being aware of past tense rules. Appropriate past tense endings for regular words are then produced which show that the child has begun to look for systematic rules in modifying words (kick – kicked, push – pushed). Mistakes may then be made on irregular verbs, even though these were used correctly earlier on (breaked, runned, buyed, eated). Later the child has to sort out which verbs are regular, when the -ed rule applies, and which irregular, when each verb will have to be learned on a one-by-one basis. It is probably true that children come to use past tense more consistently and appropriately than future tense. The immediate past is closer to the child's actual experience than things which have yet to happen, and therefore more easily understood. Whilst children are learning tense rules they may prefer to mark tense with an adverbial, before the right word endings are used: 'Yesterday, I go swimming'; double tense markings (I did rided my bike) and the missing out of auxiliaries (I been to playgroup) are commonplace.

At this stage children begin to incorporate negatives such as 'can't' or 'don't' into their sentences: 'don't bite me', 'he won't go'. In other words they begin to learn principles such as putting a negative between subject and verb. Question forms, too, become more complex and varied: 'Why you sleeping?', 'Where my Mummy?', 'What Daddy doing?' However, children still do not invert the subject and verb, which is the mature question form.

Stage IV

By the fourth stage of development, from about two and a half to three years, sentences increase to four elements of structure. Most children by the end of this stage will have acquired most types of simple sentences and commands, such as 'Mummy give that to teddy', 'Lizzie going to toddler group today', 'Me play in garden in a minute.' By now many of the rules for changing words as they are combined to express different meanings are usually mastered. Clark and Clark (1977) have described the various function words and word endings which children learn as 'syntactic glue'. A summary of the basic patterns and the sequence of their acquisition is given in table 2.1, based on Clark and Clark (1977, page 345).

In using negatives children by this stage have mastered the essentials such as 'didn't', 'nobody', 'nothing' and 'don't'. There may be a few structures still to learn and errors such as 'I not hurt the dolly' may continue for some time. In question forms children by now have mastered one important feature of the adult system: inversion of the subject and verb, as in 'Can you take me?' or 'Where are you going?' There might still be word-ending errors when question forms are used, such as 'Where my Daddy goed?' Yet to be learned are tag questions. These are forms such as 'didn't you' or 'wasn't it', which are tagged on to the end of a sentence, as in 'You read the book, didn't you?' There is still a good deal of inconsistency in the child's mastery of features such as how words are modified in use with each other, but all basic grammatical patterns are established.

Stage V

At around three years of age children begin to use complex sentences and Stage V outlines the structures which enable the child to link two or more ideas together. The earliest process to appear is the co-ordination of separate clauses by conjunctions such as 'and'. Using this device the child can connect sentences in sequence – 'We had an icecream and a ride on a donkey and Mummy got stung and …' Later on sentences may be connected with 'because', 'what', 'when', 'but', 'that', 'if' and 'so'. The child also learns to embed one sentence within another. Embedding is the process by which a preposition or adverb is used to join clauses within a sentence – 'The girl who is sitting in the Wendy house is crying'. This is often felt to be the onset of the most exciting and creative period of language development. Through co-ordination, embedding and devices such as 'but', 'so', and 'although', children are able to produce long interrelated structures. When the child is capable of extending sentence patterns indefinitely, the range of expression available to the child then has no limits.

Beyond Stage V

By three and half to four years the creative power of language has usually been realised. However, the child is still a long way from mastering the adult system. Errors have yet to be ironed out. Irregular verbs, noun forms and agreement amongst words used together, all have to be practised. Some school-age children might still produce mistakes such as 'they fed himself', 'him going home' or 'where you be running?' As the child enters school there are still many things about the grammar of English which the child continues to learn.

Some seven-year-olds persist in having considerable difficulty interpreting passive structures. Linguists have demonstrated this by asking children to play-act the meaning of a sentence using puppets and toys. Sentences such as 'Richard kissed his sister' continue to be interpreted wrongly by some children in the passive voice. 'Richard was kissed by his sister' may be acted out in just the same way as the previous sentence because the child is unaware of the shift in meaning inherent in the change in sentence structure. Many children assume, quite rightly, that the first noun in a sentence is usually the agent and not the object of the action. So, a sentence like 'The horse was kicked by the rider' will often mislead children into thinking that it is the rider who was hurt.

In school, children have a great many experiences which help them to understand different levels of meaning in words and sentences, and the relationships which exist between aspects of language in use. Many words have no fixed meaning but serve a particular function. Words such as 'it', 'on', 'who', 'but', 'that' and 'when' are used for different purposes in different sentence patterns. For example, in the sentence 'Joe is riding a bike that belongs to his brother', 'that' indicates or points to the object of the preceding clause, 'bike'. Differences between words such as 'I' and 'you' require an appreciation of relationships – that 'I' must only refer to the speaker, and 'you' to the hearer; and whilst children are always addressed by 'you' they must not call themselves that. Words like 'ask'/'tell', 'here'/'there', 'bring'/'take', 'before'/'after', and 'more'/'less' also reflect an understanding of context and demand a more subtle kind of linguistic awareness from the child.

We can only understand the child's growing sophistication in using the patterns of language structure by taking into account the richness of the child's learning experiences, through which the contrasting relationships of items like function words is made clear. Karmiloff-Smith (1978) has said that during the school years children begin to treat language as a 'problem-space' in its own right. What that means is that children continue to experiment with and think about language *for its own sake*. Knowing that there are different layers of meaning in words and sentence patterns, is of course the fount of most humour in jokes and puns. It is also the kind of awareness of language in the abstract which is required to do well on things like written tests of English usage or reading comprehension, often found in schools.

To summarise, in the normal development of grammar the basic patterns of syntax and the ability to generate long and complex sentence sequences, are established well before the child arrives in school, often by the age of three and a half years. However, the learning of grammar probably does not come to an end until late childhood as children uncover some of the subtler distinctions and ambiguities. As with phonology, knowing the stages through which ordinary children progress enables a judgement to be made

Table 2.1 *The order of acquisition of function words and word endings*

Function words and word endings		Example
Progressive	-ing	He is crying
Prepositions	on, in	The cat is in the basket
Plural	-s	Boys
Irregular past tense		Drank
Possessive	-'s	John's bike
Uncontracted copula	is	Kitty is hungry
Determiners	a, the	
Regular past tense	-ed	Jumped
Past participle	-en	It's broken
Third person singular	-s	She likes jam
Third person irregular		Does
Uncontracted auxiliary	has	She has started
Contracted copula	-'s	Baby's happy
Contracted auxiliary	-'s	He's finished
Superlative	-est	Fattest
Comparative	-er	Better
Adverbial	-ly	Slowly

about the relative maturity of one particular child's grasp of grammar, in comparison with other children of the same age.

THE DEVELOPMENT OF MEANING

We turn now to a more complex area of language located on the right-hand side of the tree diagram in figure 2.1 – the study of meaning or 'semantics'. How meaning develops alongside the child's growing competence in using words and sentences is not easy to determine. We cannot ask a very young child directly what a particular word or structure means. For that reason we have to infer how meaning grows in the course of child development. Linguists have attempted to chart semantic development in various ways, such as by counting vocabulary. In the present book we shall be highlighting the pitfalls involved when meaning is approached in a vacuum. Without doubt it is much more helpful for those who are working with children, to approach meaning through the social context in which communication takes place.

It used to be thought that a good measure of a child's increasing grasp of meaning was the number of words in the child's vocabulary. Various word counts have been made so that we have an estimate of the number of words a child of a particular age should have. A child of 18 months might have some 20 words, by two years about 300 words, and so on. There are, however, several problems with this measure. It is hard to distinguish between words that a child understands, but may not actively use in speech, and words which are used but not fully understood. A further problem is that the majority of everyday words in English, such as 'go', 'take', 'do', 'come' or 'see', have many senses. (Linguists describe these words as 'polysemic'.) So merely counting the number of separate items in a child's vocabulary will be far less revealing than discovering the range and kinds of meanings which the child has built up.

These earlier attempts to chart semantic development by counting have been called 'static' because it is assumed that every word stands for an object, event or idea, and the child simply builds up a store of meaning by adding more words. Approached in this way the study of meaning omits some very important aspects. Consider a word like 'fine'. It has several meanings which remain ambiguous until a sentence context is provided: 'I hope it's fine weather', 'He received a fine', 'fine grain', or 'I feel fine'. So, word meanings cannot be isolated from their context of use.

Furthermore, it is inappropriate to think of children acquiring words one-by-one. Early word meanings tend to be very fluid. Linguists have kept diary records of the first words children use and the first referents of those words: what the child uses them to denote. For example, one child used 'bird' to refer to sparrows as well as any other object which moved. Another child learnt 'kick' whilst propelling a ball, but also applied the word to many actions similar to kicking, such as throwing a ball. These are both examples of what is sometimes described as *overextension*. What seems to happen is that the child identifies the meaning of the word with a particular property, such as size, shape or colour. The word may then be used to refer to other objects which share the property. The word thus has a wider meaning than it does for an adult. To take another example, one child used 'scissors' to refer to all metal objects, before applying it specifically to small metal objects with moving parts, and later to implements which cut. Development consists of redefining the important semantic features.

Linguists also describe a process of *underextension*. This is where a child uses a word which seems to have a narrower meaning than it does for an adult. One child described by Clark and Clark (1977), used 'car' to refer to cars moving on the street below as she looked out of the window. She did not use the word for cars standing still, pictures of cars, or for cars she rode in herself. This child seems to have identified a highly specific property associated with 'car', and development would consist of adding to the important semantic features.

One very memorable illustration of how a word's meaning might develop has been given by Ferrier (1978). This example shows clearly how different features of a word change their significance over a period of time. On entering her daughter's bedroom every morning to encounter an offensive smell, the mother would exclaim 'Phew!' Subsequently, the child produced this word in the same setting, when there was no smell, as a greeting. Later, after 'Phew!' had accompanied some nappy-changing experiences, the child began to use the word to refer to nappies, both clean and dirty, as well as to the nappy bucket. Ferrier says that the significant features of different social contexts may be very different for adult and child and this is reflected in the different functions the accompanying language serves. For the child, 'Phew!' had a social function rather than a reference to smell. The important message here is that the word's meaning is an unstable one which has to be looked at in relation to the social situation.

The point which all these issues raise is that children's concepts about language and its meaning cannot be discussed properly outside the social context of language in use. The processes by which meanings are attached to words are active, not passive. The initial meanings which words hold are redefined and adjusted by the child until they coincide with those of the adult. This takes place as the child interacts with adult caretakers, making and testing hypotheses about the language. In order to discover how meaning develops in childhood we have to look outside the child to the linguistic interactions in which the adult and child are engaged as they negotiate with each other to reach understanding.

COMMUNICATION IN A SOCIAL CONTEXT

Whilst we can describe the sequence of stages children typically go through in their development of pronunciation, grammar and word meanings, this leaves unanswered the crucial question of *how* the child's experiences shape learning. How are children involved by their caretakers in the business of language learning? How do adults facilitate communication? How are children introduced to the rules by which conversations are conducted, such as when to listen and when to contribute? How do they master the language game in which messages are given, received, confirmed and agreed between participants? All these processes are accomplished without help by the vast majority of parents and children. Knowing what these processes are must provide some important clues for the helping process should normal development go astray.

We have said that children arrive in the world with an urge to learn more about the environment through communication. Observations of mothers and babies show that patterns of communication are established very early on, well before the child has words. Mothers deliberately stimulate the infant through singing, handling and cuddling. The child is actively engaged in social activity. The baby's burps, yawns and smiles are interpreted by the mother who will try and elicit a response – 'Have you got windy puffs?', 'Ooh that's a tired girl', 'You like that, don't you?' Schaffer (1977) has shown that the timing of the mother's stimulation is very closely tied to the child's response. For example, during feeding there may be periods of intense sucking, alternating with pauses when the mother may talk to the child. Stimulation is not simply heaped on the child. The baby's laughing, cooing and gurgling is reciprocated by the mother taking a turn to react. Many early interactions have this on/off pattern, when both mother and baby read signals in each other's behaviour. When shown a new toy the infant's visual attention or looking away will signal the child's degree of interest in the activity, which the mother may then wish to sustain or renew. Many of the early rhymes, games and jingles parents play with their infants, such as 'Ride a cock horse', or 'I can see you', encourage the child to listen to the sounds and rhythms of speech and at a critical point, the child is expected to respond in return. Researchers such as Bruner (1975) and Schaffer (1977) suggest that these early dialogues, when first the baby, then the mother responds, lay the foundations for later conversational skills.

According to Brown (1977, page 12) conversation is: 'to understand and to be understood, to keep two minds focussed on the same topic'. We can observe the mothers of three-month-old babies endeavouring to do just this, and Brown's view of communication holds true for children and adults across the age range. How, then, does the mother of a very young infant accomplish the task of keeping both minds fixed on the same target? Linguists have identified three major kinds of process which are found in the language of parents to young children. Some of these features, listed in table 2.2, have also been observed in talk between lovers, as well as to pets, plants and animals.

One kind of process serves to capture and then hold the child's attention, whilst also expressing affection. Noticeably, adults use a high-pitched, or special 'nursery' tone of voice, for talking to children, as if to signal that a child is being addressed rather than another adult. We know, too, that when recordings of adults talking to children of different ages are compared, the pitch of the adults' voices is highest to the youngest children. Adults often whisper to children and speak directly into their ears, so that it is clear they

Table 2.2   *Features of adult speech to infants*

Attention-getting	Speaking in a high pitch or nursery tone
	Whispering in child's ear
	Exaggerating intonation and rhythm
	Making use of child's name to start a sentence
	Prefacing speech with exclamation
	Special vocabulary or nicknames for child
	Touching, eye-level contact, gesturing and pointing
Simplifying	Using short sentences
	Using simple structures, avoiding complex sentences
	Omitting word endings
	Avoiding pronouns
	Selecting simple vocabulary
Clarifying	Speaking slowly and clearly
	Pausing between sentences
	Employing 'here and now' topics of conversation in familiar environments
	Providing commentary on child's play
	Using present tense
	Using more content words, fewer function words
	Repeating key words
	Providing sentence frames for new vocabulary

must listen. They also use an exaggerated intonation pattern, with rising and falling stresses. A common attention-claiming device is to use the child's name at the beginning of a sentence, such as: 'Richard, look at this picture.' Alternatively, adults sometimes preface what they say to a child with an exclamation: 'My goodness! that's a funny car.' Special vocabulary – 'dinky-doo', – provides yet another clue that the adult is addressing a child. Some attention-claiming, such as touching a child when talking, kneeling to the child's eye-level, gesturing and pointing, fall into the non-linguistic (or non-verbal) class.

A second major process observed in adult–child talk is that of simplifying – choosing the right way to say something to make sure the child understands. Adults do this by using much shorter sentences, of perhaps three or four words, to very young children. They also use much simpler sentence structures, avoiding complex sentences such as co-ordinated or embedded clauses. Certain kinds of words and word endings are omitted altogether. For example, words are shortened or given a special kind of emphasis: such as 'tummy' for 'stomach', or 'din-din' for 'dinner'. Word endings like the plural 's', or determiners such as 'the' or 'a', appear less often. Adults often dispense with all pronouns in phrases such as 'Daddy's going to put baby to bed.' Keeping vocabulary simple is another way of assisting the child. Sparrows, pigeons and seagulls are all 'birdies'. The less able the child is in understanding speech, the more the adult shortens and simplifies.

The third process in adult–child talk is that of clarifying, which also helps to ensure communication takes place. Adults speak clearly and slowly, with pauses between sentences. A lot of what the adult says is relevant to the child's 'here and now' world. Commentaries are provided on the child's play, objects are named, explanations given, relationships pointed out. Parents are skilful in talking about an object when the child is looking at it. Interaction takes place in familiar situations with familiar objects present, so the child has a good idea of what is being talked about. Present tense is more likely to be used than past or future, reflecting a concern with the immediate environment. Many more content words, such as nouns, are used, compared with function words such as 'it', 'but' or 'because'. Sentences are repeated in order to focus on key words: 'Here's your teddy. ... Get the teddy. ... Pick teddy up.' Short repeated phrases presumably make less demand on the child's memory span. The meaning may come just as easily from the play context, gestures and emphasis, as it does from the grammar. In adults' speech to children 'sentence frames' are often repeated. These are familiar, frequently used phrases which introduce new words: 'Where's the ... ', 'That's a nice ... '

When all these devices and strategies are put together, it is obvious that the spontaneous skills which adult caretakers display in talking to their infants seem designed to do one thing. They make it more likely that adult and child will share what is said and what is meant on the same topic. Adults claim the attention of children, simplify what they say, tie words and sentences to familiar objects and events, and ensure that the child comprehends through repetition. A comprehensive survey of the characteristic features of the talk of adults to infants is provided in the book by Snow and Ferguson (1977). Because of the speed with which most infants appear to learn to speak, researchers have been forced to say that the child must have some inborn facility to acquire language. This has sometimes been called a 'Language Acquisition Device' or LAD. However, it is clear from studies of adult–child talk that there are some very special features designed exclusively to help attract the child's attention, to highlight important linguistic information and to share the adult's meaning. Whatever the inbuilt capacity of the child may be, the needs of the language learner seem superbly well met in the specially adjusted behaviour of the adult.

In the Bristol child language studies described by Wells (1981), a lot of data were collected to find out how children interact with their parents at home, how they collaborate in conversation, and what strategies they use in managing to communicate. Wells proposes that the whole process of early language learning is an active one in which both listener and speaker create and search a context for clues to intended meaning. Like the Tizard and Hughes (1984) study referred to earlier, the research carried out in Bristol is one of the few projects where linguists have attempted to record the spontaneous behaviour of children at home. Wells collected language samples from 129 families using a radiomicrophone attached to the child's clothing. All that was said by the child and in the child's presence was picked up by the microphone and transmitted to a receiver, where the speech signals were recorded.

One of the most striking findings of this research is the consistency amongst individuals in the devices and strategies that are learned in order to become more expert communicators. Without the two participants in a conversation alternating in taking turns to speak, a fundamental condition for successful conversation would not be met. As we have already discovered, the rudiments of an orderly sequence of turn-taking are experienced in babyhood. Signals such as the speaker looking away for most of a turn and then looking back again when ready to handover, ensure there are no overlaps in speaking. A second strategy which makes for successful interaction is that what is said in each turn relates in part to what was said by the previous speaker, and in part to the social context in which it takes place.

Let us consider an example recorded by one of the authors as his daughter talked to her mother:

Child: I'm a mummy.
Adult: Lizzie's not a mummy, is she?
Child *(holding doll)*: Gotta baby, I'm a mummy.
Adult: Lizzie's got a pretend baby, so she's a pretend mummy.
Child: I'm a mummy, yes.

Wells (1981, page 46) says that the moves of the language game are designed around a triangle: what the speaker intends to say, how the message relates to the situation, and how the listener interprets the message. In this extract both the adult and child are talking about a doll's play context in the 'here and now'. The adult is trying to interpret what the child says and make explicit her meaning, with reference to the play situation. In fact, without the doll, which is the focus of attention of both adult and child, this dialogue would be difficult for an observer to understand. What strategies are used to sustain the conversation? Several things can be picked out. Both adult and child have obviously an 'agreement' that what they say relates to the topic in hand. Further, each contribution is linked to what was said before. In this example, pronouns and repetition link one response with another:

Child: Gotta baby, *I'm* a mummy.
Adult: *Lizzie's* got a pretend baby, so *she's* a pretend mummy.

But the adult is achieving more than this. When the child says she is 'a mummy', the adult strives to make sense of the child's intended meaning. The child gives more information using the visual clue of the doll. The adult then supplies some missing information ('pretend') to try and arrive at a mutually satisfactory interpretation. This is what Wells calls the 'negotiation' of meaning. In his terms language is a medium of interaction which can only be understood by looking beyond the words to the intentions they realise, in the situations in which they occur. We can also highlight some other skills displayed by the adult in this example. The adult uses sentences just beyond the child's in complexity, expanding and paraphrasing what the child says, whilst also providing a better sentence model: a more explicit and correct version for the child to hear. Unwittingly, then, the adult finely tunes her responses to the child's in order to facilitate a shared understanding. In chapter 5, when we consider the most facilitating environment in which children with special needs may learn language, we shall be gathering together strategies such as those displayed by the spontaneous caregiver.

LANGUAGE AND THINKING

Thinking is never more precise than the language it uses.
(Miller, 1951, page 223)

Whilst views on intellectual development in childhood have been reworked in many respects since Miller made this statement, it still holds true that *where* children take their ideas from is not easily separated from *how* children put their ideas into words. A child of one of the authors wanted to know if they would be moving house, since his mother had 'given' their address to a policeman after a road accident. This is a good example of how the child's mastery of language is closely enmeshed with active efforts to make sense of the world. Language both shapes, and is moulded by, intellectual experience.

In chapter 1 the view was put forward that language is so interwoven with the child's play, social relationships, emotional growth, thinking and reasoning, that we cannot discuss it as a subject set apart. We discussed the range of functions language serves for the child in changing and manipulating the behaviour of others. When the child arrives in school, language serves enquiry, discovery, explanation, prediction, analysis, fantasy and conceptual development. In considering the normal process of child language acquisition it is important that we tie together some of the stages we have outlined in the child's emergent grasp of vocabulary, grammar and meaning, with corresponding developments in children's growing sophistication of skills in thinking.

There will be very few teachers who are not familiar, at least in part, with the work of Piaget. According to Piaget, thinking develops out of the child's own actions in the world, not language. He believed that children discover things for themselves in play and exploration. As the child discovers new things about the environment ways are sought to express these ideas in language. But it could be said that what sets the pace in the child's urge to communicate is the *prior* discovery of important objects, people and events. Language merely encapsulates and expresses what the child has physically experienced. Piaget's theories have had a powerful influence on what goes on in primary classrooms. In particular, the idea that children should learn by direct 'hands on' experience, discovery and exploration, has led to a general acceptance of the practice that children should first *do*, and then discuss or write.

Despite the obvious influence he has had on educational practice, Piaget has never claimed that his work should be applied to teaching. His main interest lies in *epistemology*: how we know what we know, what this knowledge consists of, and how knowledge develops over time. His method of detailed discussion and questioning of children in problem situations aims to discover the nature of thinking at different points in the child's development. Thus it is the nature of logic which Piaget is charting, and not, as is frequently assumed, the nature of child development. It is important to understand this distinction, in view of some of the recent challenges which have been made to Piaget's findings.

Let us begin with Piaget's proposals on the development of logic. The core of his theory is that the processes of concept formation follow a set sequence, each stage built on the one which precedes it. At any one stage, the child has a particular logic for exploring the world, which changes as events and experiences are encountered which challenge the logic constructed. Piaget sees the child as an active explorer and the patterns of behaviour, or strategies, that the child uses to explore, are called *schemata*. Grasping an object, like a rattle, is an example of the latter. Piaget also describes two main ways through which experience is organised. Firstly, new features of the environment can be taken in by, or *assimilated* to, an existing schema. For example, if a child can pick up a rattle, the same schema can be used to grasp a doll. The second process is that of *accommodation*. Here the basic strategies, concepts or schemata, must be changed in order to cope with new situations. For example, if an object is placed out of reach the child must now crawl to reach it before grasping. Experience is always approached with the child's existing repertoire of schemata. Through assimilation and accommodation, the child's schemata gradually become more sophisticated.

In the first two years (sensori-motor stage) the child's concepts are dominated by physical explorations built on activities such as reaching and mouthing. Initially, children do not appear to distinguish between their own bodies and outside objects or events. By four months the distinction between self and other does occur, and the child will try to repeat interesting activities. Manipulating and experimenting with objects and toys, together with a growing mobility, eventually lead to the concept that objects have an independence and that the child's actions can have an effect on them. Towards the end of the period the infant begins to represent the world in symbols. When the child uses bricks to play cars, the pretend objects are assimilated into existing ideas about the world, with an important shift in that one thing can symbolise another in the child's imagination.

In the second, preconceptual, stage, from around two to seven years, the child's thinking is characterised by transductive reasoning. What that means is that children go from one particular event to another particular event to form a pre-concept. For example, one of the authors has a child who announced that it could not be night outside the house because the curtains were still open. The child sees two things which tend to occur together, the closing of curtains and darkness falling, and assumes one causes the other. Two other kinds of logic which characterise this pre-operational stage involve egocentrism and reversible thinking. Egocentrism refers to the tendency for children to see everything from their own perspective without taking in another's point of view. The child's thinking is unable to take into account all aspects of a situation simultaneously, which is demonstrated in the familiar conservation tasks. In one experiment Piaget poured water from a short, wide glass into a tall, thin one and then asked the child which held the most water. Children of three or four years, at the pre-operational stage, assume the tall glass holds most water because they focus attention on the height of the water level, even though the operation can be reversed as the water returns to the original level. Only later, when the child can take into account other dimensions, such as the narrowness of the glass, will the child be able to think logically about the conservation task.

Conservation is an important prerequisite for the thinking which characterises the third stage of concrete operations, from around seven to eleven years. Schemata such as addition, subtraction and multiplication are gained, together with the insight that these processes are reversible. The child is aware that certain properties of objects, such as weight or quantity, stay the same even when visible changes take place, as in the water jar demonstration. To do this the child has to step back from perceptual evidence and weigh the logical relationships involved. Inductive logic is also typical of this stage: the child can abstract the characteristics of objects to form generalisations or classes (such as: apples and bananas are both fruit).

The major task of the last period of cognitive development (formal operations) from age 12 years on, is to learn how to think about ideas. The child is released from the concrete 'here and now', to reason about hypothetical events with no material evidence. This kind of internal manipulation of ideas is demanded in a great many learning contexts in school, particularly at the secondary level.

It would be quite wrong to assume all that Piaget has said has been accepted uncritically. Criticism is not usually directed at the nature of logic proposed by Piaget. Rather, researchers have re-run some of the classical experiments with slight modifications, to examine the conditions under which children are able to display the level of their development in thought. For example, Piaget illustrated the concept of egocentrism in the 'three mountains' experiment in which a three-dimensional model is shown to the child. One of the mountains has a house on top, the second has a red cross at the summit, whilst the third is covered with snow. A small doll is produced and positioned to one side of the model. The problem for the child is to decide just what the doll can see. When children below six years were shown pictures of the model from different angles, they almost invariably chose the picture which represented their own point of view. Piaget interprets this as 'egocentrism': the child cannot stand back from the situation to infer another point of view.

Several investigators (such as Donaldson, 1978) feel that Piaget underestimated the importance of the conditions in which these experiments took place, to the logic displayed by the child. Donaldson describes several situations in which children as young as three years are able to see other points of view and are not egocentric in their thinking. Instead of the three mountains task, children were given a similar model involving a doll hiding from a policeman. This task also requires the child to make judgements of what can be seen from different viewpoints. The essential modification is that this new task is much more dramatically relevant to the child. The motives of the dolls and the policeman were quickly grasped by three-year-olds in this experiment who were able to make the kind of objective judgements which Piaget felt young children incapable of. Donaldson has several things to say about this. Firstly, in many Piagetian tasks, children may simply misinterpret instructions on what they have to do. Secondly, psychologists are usually guilty of giving children problems which fail to make human sense and lack purpose. Thirdly, we are all generally guilty of underestimating the young child's thinking potential. Such criticisms do not really have much bearing on Piaget's theory of logic, although they may be important to our view of child development.

Let us now consider how the development of thinking interleaves the growth of language, with further examples from other theorists as well as Piaget.

Other accounts of development, such as those provided by Soviet psychologists (Luria, 1961; Vygotsky, 1962), give a different view of the contribution that language makes to thinking. Vygotsky says that thought and speech develop along separate lines in the first two years of life. Initially, the child's speech is external and serves a social function. Later on, speech begins to serve an internal function and words become the basic structures of the child's thinking. Both Piaget and the Soviet psychologists emphasise the importance of direct experience as the child grasps, lifts, handles, and pushes objects around. However, the Soviet view is that language begins to *dominate* children's behaviour. Luria (1961) gives the example of a mother showing her child an object, such as a glass, whilst at the same time giving the word 'glass'. Luria says the word directs the child's attention to the object's essential features and makes perception of the object permanent. The word stands as a symbol for the real thing and *mediates* the child's experience. Later on the child can relate object to object using words, without needing the objects themselves to be present. The major difference between these contrasting views is one of emphasis: Piaget claims that logical thought is built on physical experience; the Soviet position is that language both facilitates and regulates thinking activity.

Whichever view one takes, the child has to advance from a state of simply reacting to sensory experiences, to one of actively categorising and organising the environment. In the very early stages, which Piaget called the sensori-motor period, the baby's explorations in looking, touching, sucking and grasping, lead to the realisation that the child's actions make things happen – hit the mobile hanging over the cot and it moves noisily. The major significance of this period of experimenting and manipulating, is that children become aware of the existence of things outside themselves. At one month the baby shows interest in surrounding objects but there is no response if an object is taken out of sight. Contrast this with the behaviour of a child of eight months or so who will search for an object hidden under a screen. The shift occurs because the child has learnt something of the permanence of objects encountered. Things exist outside the child; they can be acted upon physically; but they also can be represented as images in the child's imagination.

Knowing that objects have an identity of their own and exist even when they are hidden from view is a basic pre-requisite for language. Subsequently, objects can be represented in mental images, drawings, symbolic play, and words. The child is then poised to remember objects and events, relate one thing to another, and develop primitive categories, through mental imagery. As we have already seen, adults are adept at presenting words to children in social contexts which are relevant to the 'here and now' of the child's world. The strategies which adults use in their talk to babies are superbly well-tailored to help the child sort out the environment and draw attention to meaningful aspects of it, which can then be represented in words. What we have, then, are parallels between the child's perceptual abilities, the features which the adult highlights for the child in a social context, and the development in understanding through language, of how the world is put together.

As an illustration of how these separate influences complement each other, consider how a child's perception of patterns and shapes is reflected in the early features of meaning attached to words. One of the first objects to elicit a smile from babies is a picture of a human face. Initially, a few dots or lines suffice. Then children require a mouth to be present before they will smile, and later eyes. By five months a baby will not acknowledge unrealistic heads. Eventually, the unique patterns of individual familiar faces are recognised. The shift in perception is from individual features towards a configuration of features. The child stops looking at one particular aspect and adjusts attention to a group of important parts which make up the whole. This is, of course, exactly the sequence of development which takes place as the child acquires word meanings. A word like 'dog' may be overextended to all furry animals initially, because the child identifies its meaning with a single feature of furriness. This wider meaning of 'dog' is gradually redefined to include only four-legged creatures which bark, in line with the adult meaning. It seems likely, then, that the early semantic features which are attached to a word mirror the development of perception in the child.

What Piaget has called the egocentric way of thinking has parallels in how the child interprets and uses sentence structures in speech. Until the age of about six or seven years, two kinds of strategies are used by children in language. The first can be described as a word order strategy. Using this strategy the child assumes that all sentences follow a subject–verb–object (SVO) rule, which many sentences do. This is fine for understanding simple, active sentences such as 'Ben picked the team', but quickly leads the child into confusion when applied to sentences where the surface word order does not reflect the deeper meaning – 'Ben was picked by the team'. Presumably, children always put themselves in the main subject role, doing things to others. Later they may put other people in subject position, acting on an object. Piaget calls the stage at which children can understand logical relationships beyond the immediately apparent the 'concrete operations' stage, from around 6 to 12 years. Not until this shift away from the surface qualities of objects and their relationships occurs, will the child be able to cope with complex sentence patterns, such as 'passives'.

In the final stages of Piaget's theory, called 'formal operations', the child learns how to think through ideas, independent of a concrete 'here and now' context. As an example of abstract reasoning, consider the demands made by this sort of problem:

> The cat is asleep
> She sleeps in a box
> The box is under the bed
> Where is the cat?

Even though a child may understand the individual sentences, a special kind of deduction is required to infer where the cat is located. Deductive logic, dealing with hypothetical events rather than observing what happens, can be considered as part of the general decentring process. As we have seen, children gradually shift away from their egocentric view point, until they are able to deal with ideas in the abstract. It could be said that this kind of thinking skill is pursued throughout schooling and is valued very highly. Most children do not develop formal thinking, according to Piaget, until about 12 years, and some may never achieve it.

To take one final example from Piaget, the child's use of kinship terms like 'sister' or 'brother' shows how the gradual shift in thinking closely interacts with the use of language. A child's first meaning for 'brother' may be based on visual information – 'they look like little boys'. Later on the child adds other features such as 'they live in the same family'. However, not before the child has begun to think formally will an understanding be reached of the reciprocal relationship, that if a boy *has* a brother, then he *is* a brother.

It is a fair comment that the exact relationship between children's discovery of language and the way in which they think about the world has yet to be unravelled. We cannot say for certain whether a child has to be able to think a certain way *before* a particular language structure can be used, or vice versa. What can be upheld is the view that language and thinking both proceed by the child actively generating rules and strategies to account for experience. For those wanting to explore the area in more depth Moore and Beveridge have pursued some of these ideas further in their books (Moore, 1973 and Beveridge, 1982). The most important message for teachers, from this area of research, is that children can be stimulated by socially relevant and meaningful learning opportunities, to question, draw conclusions and make generalisations. Both language and thinking are nurtured by the child's sense of wanting to know.

Donaldson (1978, page 87) has said that the course of development is from 'an awareness of what is without to an awareness of what is within'. In other words, whilst the child's learning starts out tied to events in the immediate surroundings, eventually the child comes to turn language and thought in upon themselves. Thinking moves beyond immediate bounds to manipulate ideas, and infer relationships between objects and events, in the abstract. In the final sections of this chapter we shall be looking at two major influences on the normal child's development – the home and the school. In each case we shall be asking the question: How is the child helped to learn?

LANGUAGE AND THINKING AT HOME

The most recent opinions of writers like Donaldson (1978) suggest that in some situations, young children may be much closer in their thinking to adults than was previously envisaged. Perhaps the most compelling evidence that young children make inferences and test hypotheses, comes from the way in which children actively uncover for themselves the rules which govern the language being used around them.

For many children, almost all of these rich experiences of learning and discovery take place within the home. Parents who are instrumental in providing these important learning experiences for their child, are usually given little credit for what they do. Parents are sometimes made to feel that they know very little about children, compared with the professionally trained and qualified 'experts', such as teachers or psychologists. One commonly expressed justification for admitting children into nursery groups at the age of three years or younger, is that of giving them the sort of stimulation and experience they may be felt to be missing at home. The notion of compensatory education put forward by the Plowden

Report (DES, 1967) implies that children from economically poor backgrounds are impoverished in other ways as well. Schools are given the job of compensating for limited learning opportunities at home.

We now know that there are several respects in which these beliefs are mistaken. When researchers have gone into homes to observe what takes place, they have usually been surprised at what they find. There is a depth and intensity to children's interactions with their parents which is rarely found in schools. There are good reasons to believe this is just as true of the materially less well off, as it is of more affluent families: in this respect there are no class distinctions. How, then, do parents contribute to the development of children's thinking and language at home? What can professionals learn from parents?

We have already described some of the features of adult's talk to children which seems especially designed to signal that the child is being addressed, to hold the child's attention and to ensure that the child understands. Many strategies involve simplifying words and sentences, together with clarifying meaning through devices like repetition. There are, however, a number of other ways in which adults engage in highly productive interchanges with children which stimulate their language and thinking. Many parents read books to their children, which introduces them to the power which written language has for creating imaginary alternative worlds. They also play word games such as 'I spy' or 'I love my love with an A', and these activities are fairly obviously learning-oriented. But parents, often mothers, spend far more time with their children involved in other kinds of joint activity, such as preparing meals and doing housework. Recent evidence suggests that there is something distinctive about these ordinary social contacts at home, which provide important learning opportunities very different from those met in school.

In the study by Tizard and Hughes (1984) in which recordings were made of children's conversations at home with their mothers, one of the questions asked was 'What do children learn at home?' One striking finding was the sheer amount of talk between four-year-olds and their mothers. On average the children in the study held 27 conversations an hour. If the 'turns' in a conversation are counted, when first one person contributes, then the other, on average each conversation lasted 16 turns. Half of these conversations were started by the children themselves. At home there were few distinctions in the amount or kind of talk between working-class or middle-class families.

Talk arose out of the child's play where the adult would supply commentary, new possibilities, information and ideas, which helped the play to be extended. The range of talk covered topics such as relationships between members of the family, the size and colour of objects, time, general knowledge, history, geography, plants and animals. We suggested in chapter 1 that adults tend to believe in the 'informative' function of language (Halliday, 1975). They certainly give children a great deal of information during the ordinary course of the day. However, there is an important distinction to be made about the giving of information to children at home, compared with many school situations. At home it is more often than not the *child* who is asking for information, and the demand arises from a context in which the child has a reason to find out more. Tizard and Hughes (1984) give this example of a conversation which occurred when a four-year-old watched her mother weeding the garden:

Child: There's a dead onion.
Mother: No, they're not dead onions, they're bulbs.
Child: Are they dead?
Mother: No, they'll come up again this year. They store all the food from the old leaves ...

(Tizard and Hughes, page 39)

It is the child who instigates the discussion, whilst the adult takes the opportunity to clarify and inform in terms that the child understands. One essential aspect of this dialogue is that it stems from a shared 'hands on' experience. In the researcher's words a great many of the conversations arose 'incidentally in the course of simply living and chatting together' (page 40).

On very few occasions did the adults in this study use language to manage or direct the child (e.g. 'Don't put the cup on the TV'). Less than 28 of the mothers' 200 turns of talk per hour, on average, were of the directive kind. Adults were observed playing games like 'peep-bo', 'hunt the thimble', cards and tickling. They read stories and watched television together. They drew pictures. They went shopping and looked after babies. They planned holidays, talked about sex-roles and argued irritably together. These interactions share several characteristics. Firstly, the 'to and fro' of conversation is often sustained over long periods. Parents have the time, even when primarily engaged in a chore such as ironing, to respond to the child's questions. Every activity, including reading stories, is heavily punctuated by the child asking for clarification or more information. Since the adult and child know each other intimately, talk usually arises out of a shared context with great meaning to the participants. Many of the discussions which followed were free-ranging and referred out of context. They discussed past and future events, antecedents and consequences, cause and effect.

Tizard and Hughes (1984) pay a lot of attention to the active, enquiring demands of children at home. Very little of what the children had to say were simply statements. Almost everything required a response from the adult. On average, children in the study asked 26 questions per hour. Some of these questions were challenges – 'Why do we have to?' But two-thirds of all questions were to satisfy curiosity: how things work, where people are going, why one thing not another, what this or that means, and so on. Tizard and Hughes call the episodes of persistent questioning, through which children seek explanations, 'passages of intellectual search' (op. cit., page 114). In the following example, a four-year-old has been thinking of writing to Father Christmas about a coveted ballerina outfit:

Child: And what will he say if I write a letter to him?
Mother: He'll say, 'this looks like a nice letter, I'll see what I can get. She wants a dancer's outfit'.
Child: He won't know my name.
Mother: He will if you put your name on the bottom.

(op. cit., page 116)

Tizard and Hughes see episodes like this, where the child puzzles over inconsistencies and asks further questions to resolve them, as clear evidence of the pre-school child's logical power. Like many other authors, these researchers feel there is compelling evidence that Piaget underestimates the child's ability in thinking and reasoning, given the right opportunity to display it.

LANGUAGE AND THINKING IN SCHOOL

The learning context of the school is a different one, in several respects, from the learning context of the home. The two provide a contrasting set of opportunities in which the child can learn. Some of these contrasts are obvious. In school, children spend a lot of their time learning in groups. Adult–child interaction is perhaps less intimate than at home, with children making demands on peers more of the time and learning from each other. This is likely to affect the range and depth of interaction enjoyed by children. Peers will bring a wide set of experiences into the classroom, particularly in multi-cultural communities. On the other hand, adults who partake in conversations with children in school may share little of the child's experience outside of the classroom context. A more subtle difference between home and school is that teachers set up aims and objectives in their work: they have a curriculum to follow, a distinct purpose to fulfil. The child has to be helped to learn important skills. In some people's minds, this too has a significant influence on the kinds of interactions sustained between teacher and child.

In the early stages of school an important emphasis, particularly for children with speech and language difficulties, will be placed on enhancing normal language development, productive conversation, and using language as a means to learn. Several recent studies have looked in some detail at the ways in which adults behave in the early school years and the effect this has on language interchanges between adult and child. In the work by Wood, McMahon, and Cranstoun (1980), tape-recordings were made of the conversations between adults and children in playgroups and nurseries. Many of Wood's nursery staff behaved as managers. What they said to children reflected a concern to make sure children were in the right place with the right equipment, and that things were running smoothly:

Child: I've finished my painting now.
Adult: Oh, that's nice. Go and put it near your peg – go on, good boy. Jilly, I hope you're going to put that apron on if you want to paint. Not so much noise, please, Nigel ...

(op. cit., page 12)

This adult spent a lot of her time directing children. She did not take up the chance offered by the child to talk about her painting and there is little sustained dialogue with any of the children in the group. This finding, that children sometimes interact less fully and less frequently with adults in school, is also confirmed in the Tizard and Hughes (1984) study.

In this latter study, some children appear to come off worse than others in moving from the learning context of the home to that of the school. Particular children from the lower socio-economic groups in the Tizard study had been observed as persistent questioners at home, but were very subdued in school. The researchers felt that teachers made fewer intellectual demands on certain children, involved them less in discussion and fostered a kind of interaction where the child's role was to answer and not to ask questions. The important implication of this is that teachers need to find ways of bridging any gulf that may appear between the child's experiences at home and in school. Facilitating the child's active impulse to learn has to be a continual priority for all children, from all social backgrounds.

It is important, then, to highlight what seem to be the most productive ways of enhancing language interaction in school. The richest body of data on this issue has come from the Bristol Language Development Research Programme, mentioned earlier (Wells, 1985). Wells believes, on the basis of his extensive recordings of spontaneous conversation in homes and schools, that there is no simple relationship between language development, social class and subsequent school attainment. Wells suggests that family background is much less important in accounting for variation in language development than is the quality of the child's experiences. The key to development, Wells argues, is to be found in interaction, and this more than any other factor accounts for differences in rate of learning.

What, then, appear to be the most helpful strategies that teachers can adopt in order to interact with children in the classroom? The collective evidence of recent studies suggests that teachers are more effective in sustaining conversation when they show a genuine interest in the child, are prepared to listen to what the child has to say, and take up opportunities for talk related to the child's play and activity. The following is an extract taken from a recording by Wells (1985, page 24) of the talk between a child and her teacher in an infant class. The child has introduced the topic of 'sleeping arrangements' at home:

Child: Carol got a bed and Kelvin ... and Carol.
Teacher: Um hum. What about Donna?
Child: Donna – we're sharing it.
Teacher: You're sharing with Donna are you?
Child: (*nods emphatically*)
Teacher: Do you have a cuddle at night?
Child: Yeh an I – when I gets up I creeps in Mummy's bed.
Teacher: For another cuddle? Ooh that's nice. It's nice in the morning when you cuddle.

This is a good example of what Wells calls 'starting where the child is'. It is the child who initiates the conversation on a subject matter relevant to her. The teacher shows interest, listens, and wants to know more. The teacher's questions reveal more information, which the adult interprets, restates and expands. The conversation is handed back to the child each time and the adult waits for a reply. Comments are given from personal experience – 'It's nice in the morning when you cuddle', and a little social oil is added to sustain the dialogue – 'Ooh, that's nice'. Essentially, the adult is trying to share something of the child's world and to help the child think around her experience. Both adult and child enter the conversation as equal partners, with no effort on behalf of the teacher to correct the child's linguistic mistakes, to enforce correct responses, or to dominate the interchange. Both share a focus of interest in what the child conveys, exploring and extending their understanding of the shared topic of interest. The principles we have outlined here, for classroom talk, are built on the kind of negotiating strategies adults use with much younger infants with more limited language at their disposal. The adult's concern is to share the child's meaning, supporting and developing what the child introduces.

The evidence in favour of this kind of teacher responsiveness in relation to children's development is fairly straightforward. Children exposed to the richer kinds of interactional experience (in the terms we have described) make better progress in their learning of a first language (Barnes et al., 1983), regardless of family background. So too, children exposed to interactive styles of oral language show better educational attainments in school. Of course, other factors are important in predicting the child's success in school. In the Bristol studies, factors such as the degree to which families fostered an early interest in literacy, reading books together, helping the child to write, and generally exploring the function of reading and writing with the child, also seemed important predictors of later achievement in school (Wells, 1985).

We have said that the learning context of the school is different from the pre-school context in a number of ways. The school has an important job to do in helping children to acquire more formal ways of organising, recording, and interrogating experience. In chapter 1, we discussed some of the aims heralded by teachers and in policy documents such as the Bullock Report (DES, 1975). Schools introduce children to methods of discovering information, and ways of perceiving relationships between events. Children are helped to tease out categories; to work out how one thing stems from another; to think out the rules of a game; to choose, interpret, and consider possibilities. According to Donaldson (1978) the whole purpose of school is to enable children to make hypotheses and constructs, which can then be checked out by experience. Valued highly is the ability to reflect on things in the abstract, beyond the 'here and now'; to manipulate ideas, analyse and reflect. In this sense, the later years of school progressively use language itself as a resource. Reading, writing, and thinking about language move the child towards 'disembedded' modes of learning activity.

The theme of the child as an active discoverer in the learning process, at the hands of facilitating adults, is central to all that we have said about early language development, and applies equally well to the later evolution of language and thinking in school. The most effective learning, at all stages of education, starts from where the learner is. (Piaget would argue that children, with an 'egocentric' perspective of the world, find it difficult to start from any other point.) The teacher devises learning tasks according to the child's own purposes and level of understanding. Tasks which are simply imposed upon the child, without taking into account the child's experience and awareness, are less likely to interest the child or to develop the child's thinking. Similarly, rote learning, the mechanical rehearsal of skills out of context, such as maths tables, or phonic sounds, important as these may be, promotes a passive kind of learning, the relevance of which may be more apparent to the adult than the child.

Teacher-dominated learning, perhaps with the main aim of handing over information to the child, also runs against the grain of child-initiated learning. To use another Piagetian term, the learning ethos we have described suggests that the more productive kind of teaching challenges the child's schemata. The child is helped to reorganise an inner model of how the world works through purposeful activity. The discovery that some events and experiences do not fit into existing models and categories, encourages the child to refine the concepts held. Across the school curriculum, learning can be a joint, reciprocal partnership between teachers and children, which extends the child's understanding and fosters the kind of 'reflective awareness' which Donaldson (1978) feels is so important for intellectual development.

We shall be pursuing some of these ideas further in chapter 5 when we consider the learning context for children with difficulties in acquiring language and using language as a means to learn. Meaning-oriented strategies whereby learning becomes a collaborative, purposeful process, we shall be applying to reading and writing. Indeed, helping children to become active, independent readers, using the many clues available to discern the meaning in text, is an especially relevant approach to children with limited language under their control (Webster, 1986a). On a final note, it is hoped that this discussion of how language and thinking can be promoted in school is not perceived as being didactic. The last thing we would want teachers to feel they have to do, is to embrace strategies rigidly. Teachers who can be flexible, who will try out different approaches to meet individual children's needs, and then evaluate the success of the exercise, are best poised to decide for themselves which strategies are most effective in the classroom.

AN OVERVIEW OF NORMAL DEVELOPMENT

We round off this survey of the normal developmental process with an overview of the basic requirements and conditions necessary for language to grow. Some essential ingredients are to do with the physical make-up of the human organisms involved. We assume intact senses and a healthy brain, for example. However, we have deliberately turned our attention to the social context in which children acquire language in the company of adults. Quite simply, these are the major variables which teachers have in their control –how teaching strategies and the learning environment, rather than the child, can be modified. Figure 2.2 summarises the major factors we have considered.

For normal development to take place we must assume that the child is capable of perceiving, storing and responding to information. There are, of course, wide variations between individuals in perception, memory and thinking. Where children receive their ideas from is not easily separated from the language at the child's disposal and through which ideas are expressed. Similarly, developments in perception may shape the child's use of language. So, brain and behaviour are intimately related. It remains true that children who have damaged brains are likely to have some of these processes disrupted, such as attention, organising and retrieving information, generalising learning from one context to another, speed of learning and ability to assimilate experience. It used to be held that there were critical periods when the brain had to be stimulated, in order for the nervous system to develop properly. This may still be held; however, we know from children who have been isolated from stimulation in adverse conditions, that children's potential for learning often survives extreme deprivation.

There are some areas of the brain which are known to be closely associated with speech processing, listening and reading, such as the temporal lobe. Similarly, other areas of the brain, particularly in the brain stem or cerebellum, control the co-ordination of muscle movements. So, not only does the brain have to be capable of creating ideas, it also has to be able to plan how these ideas may be encoded in speech. At the simplest level the child has to work out how to produce and control sounds. We saw how, in normal development, the baby first enjoys a practice stage, prior to the production of speech sounds proper, when fine control of lips, tongue and the muscles involved in making speech sounds is achieved. Any difficulty which interferes with the process by which nerve impulses from the brain are translated into co-ordinated and rhythmical movements of the speech musculature, will have a profound effect on the child's communication skills.

In figure 2.2 we have made a distinction between those factors involved in producing or encoding speech, and those aspects concerned with the reception of a speech message. It is immediately

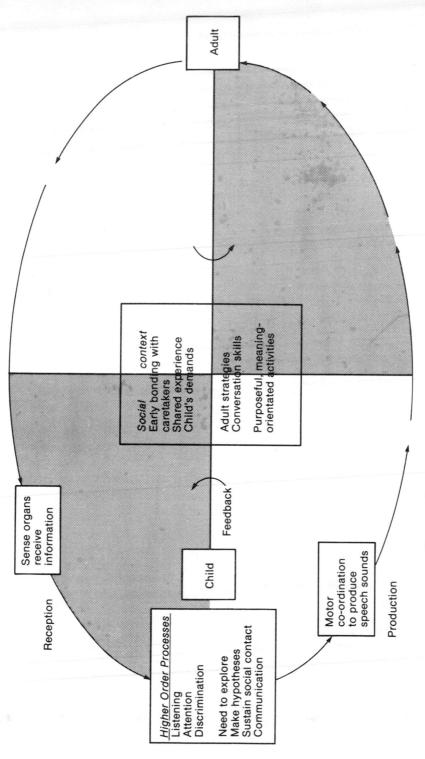

Figure 2.2 Factors involved in the normal language learning process

clear, however, that in order to encode the relevant speech sounds babies must hear the particular set of sounds used by adults around them. They have to be able to listen both to their own voices and to other people's. Deaf babies, who may receive a much more restricted and distorted auditory feedback, vocalise less purposefully than hearing babies after about six months, and may eventually stop making sounds altogether.

Good auditory discrimination is obviously a very important factor in the speech process. It is often the case that children can hear contrasts between sounds in words well before they can pronounce such contrasts for themselves. It is also often said that children are able to take in and understand language at a level more sophisticated than they themselves can express, although this may not always be the case. In other words, productive skills often lag behind receptive skills. There is nothing very surprising about this. Most teachers would expect children to be able to approach a task like reading, where there are a host of clues to the meaning, before being able to write, which involves planning and precise execution.

Auditory discrimination, then, enables children to bring their own speech production into line with the adult system as they mature. The child has to be able to detect sounds, to recognise sounds that are the same, and to differentiate small differences in sounds. In order to be able to hear sounds and to tie what is heard together with a visual or tactile experience, the child's senses have to be intact. That is an essential pre-requisite, for example, if the child is going to relate names to objects in the environment. Taking in sensory information is the beginning of what we called the reception process in figure 2.2.

Whilst children may see and hear things around them it does not always follow that they will pay attention or listen. Attention and listening are selective. They are processes which the child gradually comes to control consciously. The ability to focus attention and to ignore distractions obviously involves higher-order processes. So, we reach full circle in this chain of events. The central control mechanism of the brain is involved in responding to incoming information, selecting relevant stimuli, relating new input to what is known, sorting and categorising, making sense of the communication context, and putting together an appropriate response.

So far, we have referred to the basic physical properties of the organism which enable the child to join in the communication process. However, the features which determine whether the child learns are to be found in the social context. Observations of mothers and babies, well before the child has any recognisable words, show that the patterns for communication are established at the outset. Early turn-taking exchanges, the synchronised behaviour of the mother as she stimulates and pauses for the baby to respond, lay the foundations for conversational skills. One important ingredient for language growth, then, is a close and secure relationship between the infant and an adult caretaker.

We know that there are some very special features of the adult's speech to children which help to attract the child's attention, simplify the language input to the child and make certain that understanding is reached. We have mentioned the 'nursery' pitch and tone of voice, rhythm, special vocabulary, whispering, avoiding complex sentences and pronouns, slow speech with pauses, together with frequent repetition of key words. From the very outset, conversations between adult and child have real significance and purpose to both parties. They talk about things which matter. Adults continue to make a range of adjustments to their speech, depending on their assessment of the child's skills, in order to sustain a shared meaning. When the child is able to contribute primitive sentences to the dialogue, the adult responds by expanding what the child says, restating, interpreting, bringing in new information, and generally making explicit the child's intended meaning. The child is not overwhelmed by a barrage of complex language because the adult gauges the level of the child's understanding and carefully tailors speech complexity to the child's own.

The child is an active participant in these social interchanges with adults. The child has a drive to make sense of the world. Children test out the environment by setting up hypotheses, and then confirming or adjusting the apparent rules in the light of experience. Almost all the child's utterances demand a response. Spontaneously, many adults interact with children in a productive way. They show interest in the child's play and activity; help conversation along by supplying information and giving the child time to reply; avoid directing, over-questioning or correcting the child's speech; and stimulate dialogue by providing personal contributions. It is only when adults try to teach language by asking the child to repeat a correct grammatical form, pointing out errors and stopping the flow of conversation to repair a faulty construction, that language learning falters. It falters because the focus moves away from communication – the sharing of meaning – to the forms of language. One good illustration of this difference in approach is captured in the often quoted example, where a child announces 'I rided my bike'. An ordinary parent is much more likely to ask where the child went, rather than insisting on correct grammar.

Ultimately, the child's learning in school brings about a new emphasis, what Donaldson (1978) has called a focus on 'within', as opposed to 'without' experiences. Clearly, the learning presented through books in school requires an abstract ability, the skill of thinking about things which are not immediately present. Logical inference requires the internal manipulation of language and ideas. Children show their potential for such logical thinking early on. There are good reasons to believe that when children are involved as active discoverers in learning, collaborating with adults to discern the meaning of situations and events, then they make better progress. This is true of first language learning and can also be applied across the curriculum and at all stages of schooling. Purposeful, meaning-oriented strategies for teaching have important implications for developing literacy skills, particularly where children bring more limited speech and language skills to the learning context.

Identifying and appraising special needs

Having established a framework for understanding the normal development of language, we set out in this chapter to account for the ways in which normal processes may be disrupted. In chapter 2 we described the main dimensions of speech and language, and the sequence in which children acquire their skills. Knowing how children normally develop control over the sounds of speech, syntax and word meanings, is an important backdrop against which to consider children who give rise for concern. Teachers need to know the separate aspects of language competence, how to recognise a child with difficulties, and the point at which further advice and help should be requested.

We have deliberately tried to avoid grouping children together under medical-sounding labels such as 'dyslexic', 'aphasic' or 'dyspraxic'. We have already given some thought to the characteristics of children often 'diagnosed' in these terms. However, the medical model is not a very appropriate, or helpful, way to approach the field of language difficulty. The reason for this is that there seems to be very little that children slotted into such categories have in common. A single underlying cause for a particular language difficulty has rarely been found. The patterns of behaviour and skill displayed by a child arise uniquely in relation to the child's personality, potential for learning and environmental factors, together with any obstacles which the child has to overcome, such as a hearing loss. It follows that any attempt to help a child should be based on a careful assessment of the individual's strengths and weaknesses, rather than on a prescription for a 'known' disorder. An analogy can be drawn between grouping children with language delay for a specific course of treatment, and giving all people who complain of back pain the identical medication.

In this chapter we shall be examining those factors known to be implicated in speech and language difficulties, such as problems in hearing, vision and motor skill. We shall be looking at social factors such as the behaviour and responses of adult caretakers when they know a child has a handicapping condition such as Down's syndrome. Essentially, we shall be highlighting factors which exert a powerful influence on language growth. Where difficulties are thought to arise, we shall use the descriptive framework of chapter 2 to define them. In place of labels and categories, then, we have used descriptive parameters. Our focus is upon discovering each individual's capabilities and limitations in relation to the learning context in which children find themselves. Obvious starting points in considering factors which give rise to language difficulties are the physical sense organs such as the ear and eye.

FLUCTUATING HEARING LOSS

Mild hearing losses of a conductive nature are perhaps the commonest disorder of the sense organs found in young children. It has been said that as many as 20 per cent of primary age children suffer from conductive hearing losses at any one point in time (Murphy, 1976). This kind of hearing loss is known to be associated with a range of speech, language and learning difficulties. The reason why a mild and intermittent hearing impairment should have such a significant effect on children's progress is a complex issue, which is not yet fully understood.

Causes of mild hearing loss

Fluctuating hearing losses arise from an outer or middle ear condition which hinders the passage of sound signals across the hearing system (see figure 3.1). Conductive losses are thus due to a mechanical obstruction and are often treatable. The more severe sensori-neural impairments, where the inner ear or nerves of hearing are damaged, are not open to treatment since the hearing mechanisms are permanently harmed. Conductive problems can be caused by a hard plug of wax impinging on the eardrum, or by dried peas or marbles blocking the outer ear canal. Children with malformed ears, or a small external opening to the ear canal, may also have conductive problems. However, by far the most common cause of a conductive loss is *otitis media*. This is often associated with an infection of the upper respiratory tract, when the child has the symptoms of a cold, catarrh, runny nose, coughs and sneezes. Otitis media is the spread of infection into the middle ear via the eustachian tube. The eustachian tube connects the middle ear to the back of the nose and throat. It has the job of ventilating the middle ear space. We can feel the effects of this tube in operation when we swallow, since this opens up the tube and allows air into the middle ear cavity. We need to do this every now and then, for example in an

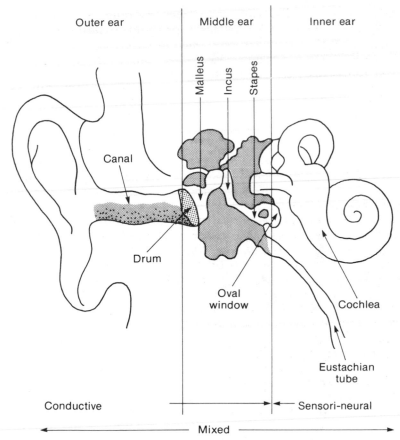

Figure 3.1 The hearing system and types of hearing loss

aeroplane, in order to equalise the air pressure on both sides of the eardrum.

If the eustachian tube is prevented from working properly through infection, a number of things may happen. If the middle ear is unventilated the eardrum will be sucked in because of the imbalance in air pressure. Stretched and taut, the eardrum will no longer be elastic enough to vibrate freely in response to sound waves. A watery fluid may fill up the middle ear space. This will affect the free movement of the tiny bones in the sound-conducting mechanisms of the middle ear. A hearing loss caused by thin fluid can come and go within a few weeks. This makes it disconcerting for teachers to decide whether a child really does have a difficulty in hearing, when the evidence for it seems to fluctuate so much. Very often children are more affected in winter months when there are more infections about. In practical terms a mild hearing loss of the order of 20–30 decibels can be likened to the effect of having one's fingers tightly plugged in one's ears.

In some children, when otitis media has gone untreated for a length of time, or when treatment has had only partial success, the middle ear fluid becomes mucoid in consistency. Thick fluid will severely dampen the signals being passed from the outer ear to the inner ear. Children sometimes have fluid in the middle ear without any symptoms of infection, such as earache, and the cause may not be known. The term 'glue' ear is often used for this condition. We have gone into some detail on fluctuating hearing loss because it appears to be increasingly common in schoolchildren, and may have significant effects on the child's development, particularly in the area of language. Unfortunately, mild hearing losses often go undetected; the child may miss or indeed *pass* the hearing screen tests in school; and it is commonplace for such children to be labelled 'lazy', 'dull', or 'disruptive'.

Identification and treatment

Whenever a teacher feels a child has difficulties in listening, concern should be shared with the parents. In table 3.1 a checklist of signs which might alert adults to the possibility of a hearing loss is provided. If there are worries, the child's hearing should always be checked out by referral to the family doctor, nurse, medical officer, or a visiting teacher of the deaf. As we have said, conductive hearing losses can be treated with medication, such as antibiotics to fight the infection, and decongestants to dry up the fluid. If the condition persists, surgery may be performed. A surgeon may draw out any 'glue' from the middle ear by making a tiny incision in the eardrum, and a 'grommet' is often inserted. A 'grommet' is a tiny plastic tube which sits in the eardrum and allows air into the middle ear. This treatment has been likened to opening a window in a damp bathroom in order to dry it out. (It can be seen from this why swimming is inadvisable for children with grommets.) It is important for teachers to realise that conductive hearing problems tend to recur, even after surgical treatment. The residual effects of a fluctuating hearing loss during infancy may well last long into the school years.

Associated learning difficulties

What are the learning difficulties associated with fluctuating hearing loss? There is fairly widespread agreement that repeated attacks of otitis media in early childhood are associated with delays in development. One of the important features of the infant's world is hearing the speech sounds of those who are around the child. If the child does not hear speech clearly, there will be marked delays in the child's own development of speech sounds, as well as immaturity in wider aspects of language. The sounds of speech most likely to be affected by a mild hearing loss are the weaker, unstressed sounds, such as the fricative 'f' or 'v' sounds, nasal sounds like 'm' or 'n', word endings and the plural 's'. Children with mild hearing losses may have problems in discriminating between sounds, in blending sounds together, and in listening out for sound contrasts in noisy conditions. A busy classroom is a noisy listening environment. It could be predicted that the child with a mild hearing loss will have great difficulty in hearing many speech sounds in the acoustic conditions of a normal school.

Some researchers have suggested that fluctuations in what children can hear confuse them at a critical time when they are processing the different sound patterns of the language (Downs, 1977). We have already discussed this idea of a critical period for language stimulation. Much of the evidence comes from experiments where conductive losses are induced in animals for a period of time and the effects observed. It is argued that reduced input in the first three years of infancy may lead to similar irreversible changes in the auditory pathways to the brain, as it does in animals. However, we know that some children do compensate for extreme early deprivation and can recover. This is true of early conductive hearing loss – children do appear to make up the early ground lost, when hearing is restored to normal.

One problem of interpretation is that factors which predispose children to conductive hearing loss, such as general ill-health, prematurity, complications during childbirth, poor environment, or family circumstances, may also contribute to delays in development. The commonsense view of this area of research is that delayed language *accompanies* conductive hearing loss. We cannot say for sure that mild hearing loss *causes* these delays in themselves. The aspects of language involved are not restricted to speech sounds. Mild hearing losses may be linked with poor auditory memory in sequencing and recalling sounds. But children may also have poorer vocabularies than normal, and a more limited use of words. They may be restricted in their understanding of words. The child's grasp of grammar may be immature, so that by the time most children are acquiring complex sentence structures in speech, the child with a hearing loss may be 12 months behind, say at stage III or IV (see pages 42–44). In school, the child may have difficulty understanding what is said, may interpret questions wrongly and be unable to put ideas into words in order to formulate a reply. As well as being poor at using grammatical structures such as plurals, different tenses, and rules which govern phrase and clause patterns, the child may also have more limited awareness of how the language is put together. This kind of insight into language as an abstract system we have described as thinking about, and experimenting with, language for its own sake. It is closely tied to other kinds of logical ability when the child stands back from immediate events to reflect and hypothesise.

To summarise, the areas of language delay associated with mild fluctuating hearing losses include the whole spectrum of linguistic skills, such as sound processing, word knowledge, and grammar, as well as deeper insights into the language system. It is inevitable that children who are less well prepared in terms of the basic language framework will also be less effective learners in school. This is exacerbated in noisy listening conditions such as a busy classroom. So, it is not surprising to find that mildly hearing-impaired children tend to be distractible, with poor concentration spans, high dependency on adults and poor motivation.

There is an extensive body of research on conductive hearing problems which has been reviewed by Webster (1986b). Some studies give test results for children who had early histories of otitis media, but no current hearing problems. On a language measure such as the Illinois Test of Psycholinguistic Abilities, children with early hearing loss tend to do less well than normal, although some studies show that the ground lost can be made up in time. Consistently, studies of children with *current* hearing loss of only 15–20 decibels (about the level of a whisper) show lower test results in reading, mathematics, and all verbal skills, compared with normal. Other researchers have looked at groups of children attending centres for remedial reading and found a very high proportion (upwards of 25 per cent) to have signs of middle ear disease. It is this last finding which should be interpreted cautiously.

Conductive hearing loss and reading

Many people have been attracted to the idea that conductive hearing loss is a detectable and treatable *cause* of reading and spelling problems. This assumption hinges on the central importance of sounds in learning to read. Obviously, if reading is introduced to children using a 'phonic' or sound-based method, the child with fluctuating deafness will find a lot of early confusions. Vowel sounds, plurals, word endings and sounds like 'f', 'th' or 'm', will be difficult to distinguish. The teacher's efforts to draw the child's attention to the links between these speech sounds and the printed symbols of the alphabet may be largely in vain. Yet we know that children who are good at categorising and recognising sounds become better spellers and readers (Bryant and Bradley, 1985.) Children who read very early, before attending school, tend to have excellent auditory discrimination. Awareness of sounds in words and having an ear for rhymes and alliteration are all important to beginning reading. Defenders of the phonic approach argue that decoding letters into sounds allows the reader to discover the meaning of a written word through hearing the corresponding spoken sounds. The child is helped to tackle new visual word patterns never met previously. If the child is a slow reader, remedial teaching geared to phonic strategies appears to help.

Despite these claims for the central role played by sounds in reading, the language model presented in chapter 2 (figure 2.1) shows the sound aspects of language and reading in a side position. Sound factors are significant in reading, but they are not the whole explanation. Very few theorists now try to explain the reading process in terms of a single factor, such as sounds. A more balanced view is that reading involves taking clues to meaning from several information sources. These might include letter sounds and shapes, recognising whole word features, and predicting meaning from the sentence grammar, together with storyline and picture clues, sensible guesswork and hypotheses based on the child's general knowledge of language and the world. As we have seen, these broader aspects of comprehension and language use cut right across the spectrum of linguistic skills, and are often affected by fluctuating hearing loss. So, there are firm reasons for suspecting a much more diffuse relationship between hearing loss and reading difficulty, over and above a specific problem in relating letters to sounds. (For further discussion of the wider developmental issues involved in both reading and deafness, see Webster, 1985a.)

SENSORI-NEURAL HEARING LOSS

So far we have discussed the implications of mild hearing losses for the development of speech and language. It is important for teachers to realise that there may be two or three children in every primary classroom who suffer a fluctuating hearing loss and this is likely to be associated with a wide range of speech, language and learning difficulties. Fortunately there will be only two or three children in every 5000 who have more severe deafness as a result of permanent damage to the nerves of hearing (Webster and Ellwood, 1985). However, of all the factors known to contribute towards communication difficulties, a severe sensori-neural hearing loss has perhaps the greatest impact.

Causes of sensori-neural deafness

Sensori-neural deafness usually stems from damage to the inner ear or auditory nerve pathways to the brain. Some children inherit deafness. Other prenatal causes include damage to the inner ear through a viral infection, such as influenza, contracted by the mother during pregnancy. If a mother has German measles during the third or fourth month of pregnancy there is a high risk of the baby being affected. The rubella virus can lead to a number of defects in the child, such as blindness, heart or brain damage, or deafness or a combination thereof. For this reason, teenage girls in the United Kingdom are immunised against rubella and therapeutic abortions are offered to mothers known to have had rubella at a critical time in pregnancy. A few years ago an epidemic of German measles meant a certain increase in the numbers of severely hearing-impaired children, and people must be guarded against complacency over immunisation.

Some severe hearing problems are caused during the time of birth, perhaps as a result of a long and complicated labour. This is sometimes due to lack of oxygen which results in damage to the nerve cells in the auditory pathway. Premature babies are more likely to be injured during birth, to contract infections and to suffer lack of oxygen. Other conditions which may affect the newly-born child include jaundice, caused by a mismatch between the blood groups of the mother and baby, which damages the nerves of hearing. The commonest postnatal cause of deafness in young children is probably meningitis. This is an acute inflammation of the covering of the brain which can lead to spasticity and mental handicap, as well as hearing impairment. Occasionally, childhood illnesses, such as mumps, measles and chickenpox, lead to deafness, although the severity of the primary illness may not necessarily have been great.

Identification and diagnosis

Because the effects of deafness can be so devastating, efforts are made to identify hearing losses as early as possible in children, through the community health service screening programme. Health Visitors test every baby around the age of eight months to see whether the baby responds to everyday sounds. In some areas the parents are asked to complete a questionnaire which gives them an opportunity to register any worries they might have about their

Table 3.1 *Warning signs of a hearing loss*

Medical records or siblings show a history of ear infections or failed screening tests, especially in winter.
Frequent coughs, colds and absences from school.
Complaints of earache, 'popping' ears, catarrh, or visible discharge from the ear.
Immature speech sounds, with some word endings omitted, and confusions between similar sounding words.
Louder or softer voice than is usual, mouth-breathing, snoring.
Limited vocabulary and immature sentence patterns.
Appearance of better hearing when speaker's face is visible, with facial and lip clues.
Slow response to simple instructions or questions with inappropriate responses made.
Continual pleas for repetitions of spoken word, or following of other children's lead in carrying out class instructions.
Misunderstandings if a sequence of instructions is given.
Turning of head to locate a sound or to give one side an advantage.
Need to sit nearer a television than is usual or requests for volume to be turned up.
Daydreaming, drifting off, withdrawal, little part taken in discussion or conversation.
Inattention, distraction of others, greater response in quiet conditions or small groups.
Irritability and atypically aggressive outbursts, more frequent upsets in school.
Inability to follow a story especially in noisy listening conditions.
Failure to turn immediately when called by name, unless other visual clues are given.
Tiring easily, poor motivation, listlessness, lack of energy, difficult to reach, stress signs such as nail-biting.
Particular school difficulties in verbal areas such as reading, 'phonic' work, writing; may be much better in practical subjects.
Periodic falling away of learning and attention with greater demands for individual help.

child's hearing. Children are usually given a hearing screen test when they start school at five years of age. Whether or not a child has passed a screening test, or has medical records which declare normal hearing, if an adult who knows the child feels worried about that child's hearing, then it should be checked out. Teachers in school should be alert to the likely symptoms of hearing loss given in table 3.1. Every now and then children escape detection, despite severe hearing problems, until school age. A child in school may suddenly acquire deafness in one ear or both, following a viral infection. The onset of a hearing problem could produce symptoms such as lack of attention, poor concentration, tiredness, listening difficulties, behaviour upsets and a fall-off in performance. Any concerns about hearing should immediately be shared with parents, the school nurse or medical officer, family doctor, or a visiting teacher of the deaf. In some areas parents can refer themselves to a hospital audiology service.

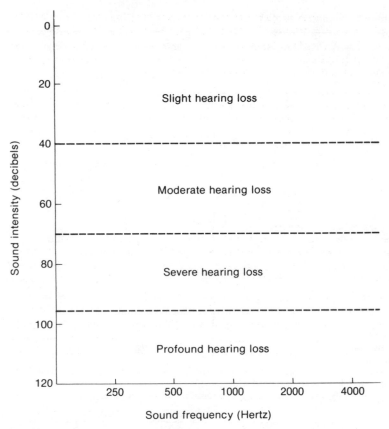

Figure 3.2 Audiogram showing categories of hearing loss

It is the job of the audiologist, using a range of highly sophisticated techniques, to ascertain whether a child has a hearing loss. The ENT specialist attempts to diagnose the nature and cause of deafness and whether any treatment is required. The results of a hearing test are sometimes displayed on an audiogram (figure 3.2). This gives an indication of the different levels of sound the child can detect at different frequencies. In other words, we discover how loudly sounds have to be made across different pitches, from high to low, in order for the child to hear. The further down the audiogram a child's hearing thresholds are recorded, the greater the hearing loss. As a help in interpreting an audiogram a whisper is around 20 decibels and the sounds of normal speech are around 50 decibels. So a child with a 20 decibel loss would not hear a whisper and the child with a 50 decibel loss would be unable to hear normal conversation.

A jet aeroplane at close quarters creates about 120 decibels of noise. A child with a 120 decibel loss would, therefore, be unable to hear a jet aircraft. Sensori-neural losses are usually uneven across the frequency range. Typically, a child may hear better at low frequencies than high, and there may be discrepancies between the two ears. This contrasts with a conductive hearing loss where the child's sensitivity to sound is usually dampened, showing a flat loss across the frequency range. Some children have both sensori-neural and conductive deafness, which reduces the child's hearing sensitivity further still. The audiogram shows hearing for pure tones and this is only one aspect of audiometric testing. However, it is the pure tone audiogram which teachers are most likely to come across in the child's records.

Treatment

It is, sadly, the case that medical science has no available treatment for sensori-neural deafness. Damaged nerves of hearing cannot be repaired. Often the only significant 'treatment' is the provision of hearing aids. Hearing aids reduce the impact of deafness at source. They do not *restore* a child's hearing to normal in the way that spectacles compensate for poor vision. They simply make sounds louder. If a child has a profound hearing loss, the most powerful hearing aids may not provide much useful sound information to the child. Nevertheless, there are very few hearing-handicapped children who derive no benefit at all from hearing aids. Most people are unaware of the problems children have in listening through hearing aids. Hearing aids pick up all sorts of unwanted sounds which are amplified into the child's ear and interfere with what the child really needs to listen to, such as the teacher's voice. The effects of a serious hearing loss, even when the child is provided with efficient hearing aids, are often overwhelming.

Developmental difficulties

It used to be thought that the main problem for deaf children is that they are cut off from the ordinary speech environment. When a child cannot hear speech clearly, even wearing powerful hearing aids, there will be enormous difficulties in acquiring basic language skills. One consequence for the deaf baby is that the vocalisations of the early stages gradually tail off and lose purpose, because the infant cannot hear surrounding speech. The child's hearing loss affects the phonetic characteristics of speech sounds as they are perceived and produced. We do not, as yet, fully understand how the mechanisms of speech perception relate to other aspects of language development, such as sentence structure. However, if a child cannot hear the important phonemic contrasts, there are likely to be delays and confusions in acquiring vocabulary, word structure and syntax. Research evidence has begun to show that deafness does not simply limit or distort what the child can hear. In fact, the child's language development may be disrupted well before the emergence of speech sounds. It will be recalled that the very first adult–child interactions such as turn-taking, mutual eye contact, and dialogues, when first mother and then baby responds, have a definite purpose. They are the first 'conversations' about a shared experience, the roots of communication. When observations have been made of mothers interacting with their deaf babies, turn-taking games, mutual eye contact and mother–infant voicing, seem to be interfered with, or missing altogether (Gregory and Mogford, 1981).

When parents know their child cannot hear, something curious may happen to the spontaneous behaviour of the adult. We have described a number of strategies which can be observed when adults talk to young children, designed specially to secure children's attention and to ensure the message is understood and meaning shared. Without being conscious of it, parents naturally tailor their sentence complexity, use repetition to highlight key words, paraphrase and expand upon the child's intended meaning, and generally *foster* the child's own discovery of language. Perhaps because parents' expectations of deaf children are less optimistic, some of these intuitive skills seem to be lost. Parents occasionally feel it is not worth talking to the child, since the child cannot hear. On the other hand, some parents feel they have to compensate by flooding the child with talk and deliberately trying to teach the names of new things. Certainly, the rich interaction and 'negotiation' of meaning readily observed in adult–child talk is conspicuously absent. In Gregory's (1983) recordings of mothers' speech to their three-year-olds, mothers of hearing children were observed *discussing* a set task with their child, such as how to go about shutting the door. Mothers of deaf children tended simply to *give commands*. Language delay is attributed not merely to the children's limited auditory experience, but also to less nurturing adult–child interactions.

It has already been noted in chapter 1 that the labels we use to categorise children can colour teacher-expectations. For example, if it is widely believed that a profound hearing loss prevents children from learning to speak, the teacher will lower the demands made upon the child and anticipate problems even before they arise. The strategies which teachers use in school to sustain conversation can be either productive or negative (Wood and Wood, 1984). When teachers give personal contributions, involve the child in conversation, allow time for response and provide 'social oil', then interaction is sustained and the child is an active participant in the learning process. On the other hand, adults who try to teach language through questioning, asking for corrections and repetitions of model sentences, tend not to stimulate language because the learning experience becomes passive and rote. Put simply, the more degree of control the teacher exerts over a conversation, through directing and interrogating the child, the less productive talk will be. In the following extract taken from a text book on the teaching of language to deaf children, it is quite obvious that the teacher's concern is with the grammatical correctness of the child's sentences, with little regard for what the child is trying to convey:

Teacher: Why do you like nice weather?
Child: Because ... because father and mother, father and mother, brother and I go swim!
Teacher: Say it better.
Child: Because father and mother, brother a ...
Teacher: Brothersss ....
(interrupting)
Child: Brotherss and I ... go for a swim.
Teacher: That is right!

(Van Uden, 1977, p. 265)

We should not make the same mistake ourselves of assuming that all hearing-impaired children are the same, have similar obstacles to overcome in learning, and always end up with limited achievements. Hearing-impaired children should be approached as individuals. The methods which are used to help children should not be rigidly applied. Some children and their families are helped to overcome communication difficulties by the introduction of a signing system early on, whilst others would prefer to use speech; opinions differ likewise amongst professionals who advise the families. No one teaching method can guarantee success and we need to be flexible. It should be noted that the majority of deaf children (more than 90 per cent, according to Meadow, 1980) have hearing parents, and their initial exposure to language is through spoken English. The circumstances of deaf children with deaf parents, whose cause of deafness is usually genetic, are very different. In many deaf families children are introduced to sign language as the primary medium of communication. There is evidence to suggest that in the latter situation, deaf children are likely to encounter fewer emotional disturbances or behaviour problems, but may make better progress in reading and academic achievement. There is a difference of opinion as to whether deaf children of deaf parents speak less intelligibly than deaf children born to hearing parents (Quigley and Kretschmer, 1982). In deaf families a strong case can be argued for 'mother tongue' teaching of spoken English through sign, in the same way that mother tongue teaching might be recommended for bilingual children in order to foster fluency in the home language and as a medium for instruction.

Deafness and language learning

What kind of learning difficulties does a severe hearing loss present? Quite apart from the interference in early patterns of social interaction with parents and the tendency for teachers to take control more, deafness also disrupts other learning situations. In school the child is unable to overhear the interactions and discussions of others. Because of the stresses of listening through hearing aids, and the need to be face to face with teachers, a great deal of information may be missed. Language is learned in the 'to and fro' of conversation as the participants make contributions and gauge the reactions of others to what is said. A child usually arrives in school with a sophisticated vocabulary, language structure and range of concepts. The child already has a framework for dealing with experiences, relating new information to old, and for thinking imaginatively about past or future events. For the severely hearing-impaired child of school age a pattern of immaturity across a wide range of language skills may be found.

At the sound level, we can attribute problems in mastering the sound system to the incomplete auditory information and feedback received by the child, even when hearing aids are worn. Vowel sounds may be distorted, consonants and word-endings omitted, speech rhythms slow and laboured, with poor breath control (see summary in Ingram, 1976). As a result, to an untrained listener, the severely deaf child's speech sounds may not be intelligible without knowing something of the context. In a study by Markides (1970), untrained listeners were asked to assess the speech intelligibility of deaf schoolchildren and only 19 per cent could be reported correctly. In the study of deaf children's speech by Dodd (1976), 11-year-olds were using about half of the 40 or so distinctive sound units of English and these had been acquired very slowly. An intriguing suggestion has been made by Conrad (1979) that children require *inner* speech sounds, spoken sounds used covertly when reading or thinking, in order to make progress. It has been argued that if deaf children do not have these inner speech-like experiences they are unlikely to become good readers and to handle long sentence sequences. The same comments can be made here as were made about the role of sounds in the reading problems of children with mild fluctuating losses. Sounds are but one aspect of language and reading, and there are many more factors involved, including the ability to think about language in the abstract (see Webster, 1985b, 1986a).

At the grammatical level, studies of severely deaf children show that early development is similar to normal in some respects, albeit delayed. For example, when deaf children are exposed to sign language as infants, the stage of 'overextension' can be seen. The child may use a sign such as 'more' to indicate a range of meanings – 'more apple', 'more sock', 'more play'. However, a deaf child is likely to acquire words more slowly and the different stages of syntax development appear later than normal. In Gregory's (1983) study, for example, a group of profoundly deaf children had less than ten words at the age of four years. By school age, some severely deaf children may be using the sentence structures of a hearing two-year-old at Stage II. Whilst deaf children continue to make progress in using grammar throughout the school years, the range of complex sentence structures mastered by hearing children at Stage V and beyond may cause problems for many deaf adults. There is one particular aspect of the grammatical competence of deaf individuals which is typical of much younger hearing children and some language-disordered children. This can be described as a word order strategy – an assumption that all sentences in English follow a subject–verb–object pattern. This strategy is fine for handling simple, active, declarative sentences such as 'I've kicked the horse,' but quickly leads to misinterpretation when applied to more complex structures, such as passives, where the surface word order does not reflect the underlying, deeper meaning – 'Joe was kicked by the horse'. In chapter 2 we discussed this strategy in terms of Piaget's views of egocentric thinking. Indeed, deaf children are often characterised as being rigid and unable to see other people's points of view, which neatly demonstrates how pervasive the influence of a child's linguistic development may be, in relation to personality and behaviour.

Some of the semantic features of language are not fully mastered by deaf children until much later than normal. This is particularly clear in children's use of metaphoric language. A deaf child may have learnt the literal meaning of the word 'time' in the sense of 'What time are we having tea?', but be totally confused by expressions such as 'take your time', or 'have a good time'. Prepositions in sentences such as 'on the bus', 'in the water' or 'by the road' may cause few problems, unlike the less literal meanings of 'on Friday', 'in the end', or 'by autumn'. It is part of the richness of

English that nuances of meaning are acquired as language is used in a multiplicity of contexts. For the deaf child, restrictions in linguistic experience may result in a confused understanding of expressions such as 'hammering on the door', 'my heart bleeds', 'shut up shop', 'dig your heels in'.

Reading, writing and deafness

A comprehensive study of the syntax of deaf children aged from 10 to 19 years has been carried out in the USA (Quigley and Kretschmer, 1982). They found that certain types of sentences, such as embedded structures, were not understood. When given these two sentences to read:

> The boy kissed the girl
> The boy ran away

most students understood them, but when given

> The boy who kissed the girl ran away

believed it was the girl, not the boy, who ran away. When deaf people are unable to use complex sentences, a large gap opens up between the level at which deaf individuals think, feel and imagine, and the level at which they can express themselves. This is precisely what is happening to the child who wrote this piece:

> Last Saturday I went to shop. I stared the boys gang were fighting. I laughed the boys they dyed their hair green. I want skinhead but I can't skinhead because my ear mould. The people see my earmould. I am embarrassed. I want to boxing. My mother said 'I'm not having it'. I was be better fighting because my hands is strong. They boys be frightened to me.

This profoundly deaf 16-year-old boy, of good intelligence, has some real adolescent feelings about wanting to be tough in the eyes of a gang of skinheads. Sadly, reality intrudes in the form of his mother's restrictions, and embarrassment over earmoulds. We feel the pressure of what this lad wants to say bursting out of the language structures at his disposal. Some features of this piece of written work are held to be typical of deaf children. There are many errors and omissions, particularly of function words – 'They boys be frightened to me'; and sentences tend to follow a rigid pattern – 'I want ... ', 'I stared ... ', 'I laughed ... '. When he tries to attempt a more complex verb phrase he goes wrong – 'I was be better fighting' – and one has the feeling that he has so much to say that he dispenses with formal grammar to organise his thoughts and just simply puts the important words near together –'I stared the boys gang were fighting.' Because some of these language patterns are so unusual, and certainly not observed in the writing of hearing children, the language of people who are deaf is considered to be both delayed and *deviant*. The devices that children normally use to create and extend their sentences, such as co-ordination using 'and', are largely missing, although the 16-year-old quoted above does attempt to use 'because'. Notice that there are no spelling mistakes, a point we shall be returning to in chapter 5 when we consider ways of helping children. The spelling skills of deaf children have important implications for the teaching of spelling generally.

Both reading and writing are skills which many severely hearing-impaired children find hard to master. Most hearing children bring to reading a sophisticated mastery of spoken language. They meet vocabulary, sentence patterns and concepts, with which they are already familiar. Faced with reading, the deaf child may not only have to learn the written symbols of print, but also the words and sentence structures which the print represents. Learning to read therefore becomes a language-learning process too. To understand the literacy problems of those who are deaf we have to look beyond the simple fact that a child may not be able to hear the sounds of letters in words. Deaf children have no problems remembering the visual patterns of words, which is why they are often proficient spellers. Reading and writing difficulties usually begin when children attempt to understand, use, and think about sentence patterns outside their control.

This aspect of reading is not exclusive to the severely hearing-impaired. A problem for all children who experience language delay arises when they meet up with a language in books which is overwhelmingly more complex than their own. There are some important principles for 'remedial' work here, which we shall be enlarging on in chapter 5. How do we help a child make sense of the complex language of reading books? One thing we can do is to capitalise on the child's natural hypothesis-testing approach to language generally. We can help children make better use of the limited language skills at their disposal (Webster, 1985b).

To summarise, a severe hearing impairment interferes with a wide range of developmental processes. From the outset, patterns of behaviour such as mother–child interactions are disturbed. Adults may behave in more directive and controlling ways as they try to 'teach' language. These secondary effects of deafness contribute to delays in a wide range of language skills. Sounds, grammar and concepts may be very delayed and in some respects deviant. There may be accompanying immaturities in social adjustment, emotional development and relationships with peers. When the child comes to school, reading and writing present large hurdles and require learning strategies to be very carefully thought out.

VISUAL IMPAIRMENT

Vision is just as crucial to healthy child development as hearing and is also involved, though less obviously so, in normal language acquisition. There is, of course, a continuum of visual loss with some children at one end with mild short-sightedness whose impairments are corrected by glasses. At the other extreme, a very few children, perhaps about ten per cent of those described as 'registered blind', have no sight at all. So the picture of total darkness evoked by the word 'blind' is inaccurate. Most visually-impaired children have some vision and the whole thrust of education for this group of children is towards using residual vision to the full. In the present context it is important that teachers know something of the causes, symptoms and learning obstacles associated with visual loss, particularly in relation to the likely effects on communication. (See Chapman and Stone, in this series, for a detailed account of visual impairments and their educational implications.)

Causes of visual impairment

Various diseases and conditions give rise to visual loss. Some abnormalities, such as cataracts which cloud the lens of the eye, are inherited. Mothers exposed to German measles early in pregnancy run the risk of having a baby with a serious visual handicap, as well as hearing and heart defects. Other conditions arise in the period surrounding the birth. At one time a number of premature children suffered visual impairments through being given too much oxygen at birth. This condition, known as retrolental fibroplasia, causes abnormal growth of the blood vessels at the back of the eye and damage to the retinal cells. A number of children lose their sight through accidents or disease, such as a tumour on the optic nerve. Serious visual defects often do not occur in isolation and may be part of a complex of disabilities.

The majority of eye conditions in children are not seriously handicapping. Spectacle wearers in school are often children whose vision is impaired because of *refractive* problems to do with the shape of the eyeball. The short-sighted or *myopic* child can see near objects better than far. This results from an oval shaped, over-long eyeball, which causes light to be focussed in front of the retina rather than on it. Far-sightedness, or *hypermetropia* means that the child can see far objects better than near. In this case the eyeball is too

Table 3.2 *Interpreting the Snellen measures of visual acuity for corrected vision*

Snellen measure	Interpretation
6/6	Normal distance vision
6/9	Mild loss
6/12	Child needs to sit near a visual display
6/18	Lowest acuity for blackboard work
6/36	Considered partially-sighted – will require low-vision aids and special text
6/60	Very limited vision
3/60	Registered blind – sighted methods inappropriate

short and light focusses at a hypothetical point behind the retina. *Astigmatism* is another common problem caused by an oddly shaped lens leading to blurring of certain parts of the visual field. Squints result from poor muscular co-ordination between the eyes and can lead to the vision in one eye being suppressed by the brain.

Identification and treatment

The routine medical and community health screening of babies, infants and school children are likely to identify most of the major visual handicaps. Children's vision is often ascertained using the Snellen charts, which measure distance acuity. The child is asked to read a list of letters of gradually decreasing size. Depending on how far away from the chart the child stands and the size of letters which can be seen, visual acuity is described as a fraction. The upper figure represents the distance from the chart, the lower figure the size of the letters: 6/6 vision means the child can see the smallest letters at six metres, which is normal; 6/60 means a child can only read the largest of the letters at six metres. A child with normal vision would be able to detect the largest letter from a distance of 60 metres away. In table 3.2 some rule-of-thumb interpretations are given of different visual acuities with the best correction possible, for example, wearing glasses or contact lenses. It should be noted that the Snellen measure does not take into account some other visual defects such as colour blindness, tunnel vision, or deterioration in parts of the visual field. However, the Snellen fraction is widely found in children's records and teachers need to be able to interpret it.

Teachers can be alert to a number of signs which sometimes indicate a visual impairment. Children whose eyes turn or squint, who close one eye to look, who rub, brush or screw up their eyes may have a problem. Unusual head postures, peering, tilting the head, eye-poking and holding reading material at odd distances or angles are symptomatic. The child may be clumsy in moving around and tend to walk with hands at the ready or outstretched. Difficulty in copying from the blackboard and books, poor hand–eye co-ordination, and large or spidery handwriting, should be noted. Children with a visual loss may tire very easily, show a lot of distractibility and make poor progress in areas such as reading. Children with visual impairments do not know that others see things much more clearly and therefore will not complain about the details they miss.

When a teacher has become concerned about a child's eyesight, parents should be consulted and referral made to the school nurse, school medical officer, family doctor, or the ophthalmic department of a local hospital. A visiting teacher for the visually-impaired will be able to assess the implications of a visual loss, what the child can cope with in the classroom, and any additional help required. In many cases, spectacles will enable the child to join in the normal learning experience. The teacher should ensure that glasses are kept clean and worn at all appropriate times. A child's visual capabilities can change markedly over time and it should not be assumed that because a screening test was passed some years earlier the child therefore has good vision. Some eye conditions require medical treatment, whilst in other children vision is permanently damaged.

Language and visual loss

Well before the onset of speech sounds and words, children come into contact with their social world. In chapter 2 we stressed the importance of these early social interactions for communication. The mother deliberately stimulates the child, and through smiling, eye contact and mutual response, the infant is engaged in important reciprocal 'language games'. One of the features of early interaction which Bruner (1975) highlights is the importance of mutual gaze as the child and adult share a visual experience together, which provides an opportunity for the adult to tie words to important objects or events. When vision is impaired these early processes are dislocated. Quite apart from the emotional disappointment when the mother cannot establish eye contact, or make the child look and respond, the child may be unable to see the mother's expressions and gestures. This sharing of experience depends on the child being able to see the focus of interest. If vision is impaired the child lacks an important dimension.

In the early period of 'sensori-motor' intelligence, to use Piaget's term, the child becomes aware of objects and events in the environment primarily through visual and tactile exploration.

Reaching and grasping; the urge to become mobile; exploring space; coming to know that objects exist outside oneself and are permanent, even though hidden from view: all these discoveries about the world are much harder to achieve with low vision. The main language difficulty associated with visual impairment is therefore a *conceptual* one. Children may have problems recognising things presented to them, in making hypotheses about relationships between objects, in identifying people, forming categories, and generally knowing what stands behind many word meanings. This characteristic has been called the 'empty language' of the visually-impaired.

John, a seven-year-old with a severe visual impairment from birth, accompanied much of his play with appropriate language – e.g., 'I'm going to bump you with my car' (pushing large trolley). At times John repeated phrases that he 'parroted' with no relevance to current activity – e.g., 'Is John going to have a honeyed cracker?'; 'What a good boy John'; 'Are you just going to lie there?' He also found many confusions in mapping meanings from one word to another. He learnt what a car 'horn' did, and then asked which of a cow's 'horns' was responsible for the 'moo'. The following conversation illustrates the features of everday experience that may be salient to the visually-impaired child and the superficial understanding that may arise:

John: *Putting the dishwasher on*
Adult: *What does it do?*
John: *Buzz*
Adult: *What do you put in the dishwasher?*
John: *Pyjamas*

Visual problems create difficulties for exploring and interacting with the world, linking words with objects and tying concepts and categories to the environment which they represent. Many visually-impaired children may show delays in acquiring language skills. At the sound level it has been argued that children around the age of six months watch mouth shapes and copy lip movements from adults. There is some evidence that a child who cannot see well may have problems in using some speech sounds, particularly those which have a clear lip pattern such as 'm' (Mills, 1983). However, as we discussed earlier, many of the speech sounds are indistinct visually, so it is more likely that speech sounds are delayed as part of an overall language immaturity. Certainly, many visually-impaired children are reported to have fewer words than normal and to take longer to acquire sentence structures. There may also be differences and delays in the child's development of meaning in language. Clearly, distant objects such as birds, aeroplanes, rooftops and ceilings, together with the language of space, colour and movement, may have different associations for the visually-impaired.

At home, especially in the early stages, a child's experience will need to be enriched by introducing a variety of sensory stimulation – sounds, smells, textures and shapes. Parents will need to accustom themselves to accompanying their everyday activities, such as making the dinner, with verbal descriptions of what they are doing. In order to avoid an echoic 'parroting' of language, what the adult says must be locked into the child's experience and environment. In school, a child's visual difficulties may be highlighted for the very first time in relation to written materials. The child's learning difficulties in school are to do with *access* to the traditional ways of presenting and recording information. When allowances are not made for blackboard work, small or indistinct text in books, or materials which glare, shine, or have too many colours and details, then the visually-impaired child may fall behind. In writing there may be confusion over similar letter shapes and difficulties keeping the place in a text when copying. With better lighting, magnification aids to enlarge small print, tactile letters, and reading materials with clear print and illustrations access to learning can be greatly improved. (For further discussion see Chapman, 1978.)

PHYSICAL DIFFICULTIES (See Lonton and Halliday, in this series, for a more detailed account)

There is a tremendous range of physical disabilities which may affect children and give rise to language difficulties. We shall make two very broad distinctions in relation to physical disability. In the first place there are children who have normal muscles and limbs, but whose higher order 'control' mechanisms are defective. In other words, the brain fails to send correct signals to the outlying parts of the body which have to be moved in co-ordination with each other. The locus of the problem, therefore, lies centrally in the brain or spinal cord, rather than in the limbs or muscles themselves. A child's loss of voluntary control may be mild and affect just hand movements. In a severe case the child might be unable to stand or walk. The physical movements necessary for normal speech can be interfered with in a child whose motor co-ordination is only mildly affected. Whenever a child suffers gross motor difficulties there are almost certainly going to be associated speech and language problems.

The second broad category of physical disability which can affect children's development includes all those conditions where there is a problem in the bones, muscles, organs, and limbs themselves, rather than in the 'control centre' of the brain. Perhaps the clearest example of a structural defect which interferes with normal speech and language growth is a cleft-palate. Children with a palate deformity may be unable to control the movement of lips and palate necessary to produce speech sounds properly. The locus of the problem is specific to the area of the ear, nose, and throat. In this case the brain sends the correct signals to the speech musculature, which is operationally deficient.

Needless to say, the wide range of physical conditions in these two broad categories are caused by an equally varied and wide range of factors. Some conditions, like cleft palate, can be inherited; others arise because of adverse circumstances surrounding the birth; whilst other conditions are acquired as a result of disease or accident.

Cerebral palsy

Damage to the central nervous system, that is to say, the spinal cord or the brain, can lead to one or other form of cerebral palsy. Sometimes, the cause of this condition is unknown. Occasionally, cerebral palsy is related to a viral infection or disease during pregnancy. Brain damage can result from lack of oxygen supply to the baby due to a twisted umbilical cord or the placenta becoming detached. Prematurity, birth injuries or a difficult delivery, are also associated with cerebral palsy. Brain damage may also result from mishaps, such as a road traffic accident.

Whatever the cause, the symptoms of cerebral palsy are produced by damage to the areas of the brain which control movement centrally and send nerve impulses to the muscles. The child may have very rigid limbs and exaggerated movements. This is sometimes described as 'spasticity' when some muscles are weakly contracted and others contracted too much. Spasticity may affect just one side of the body, or involve different combinations of limbs. In other conditions the child shows very floppy, unco-ordinated movements. Some children are unsteady on their feet and have difficulty in balancing and a very ungainly walk. Other children have more specific problems, perhaps in negotiating 'fiddly' tasks like fastening buttons, tying shoelaces and controlling a pencil.

When a child's apparent co-ordination problems are very mild it becomes difficult to determine whether there is, in fact, an underlying physical defect in the central nervous system. All children start out in life with immature motor skills which are developed and controlled as they grow. Not until the age of about two and a half years can most children be expected to have achieved co-ordination of large muscles involved in running, jumping and mounting stairs. Similarly, the fine motor skills expected of a three-year-old in picking up and manipulating small objects are very different from those expected of a one-year-old with a more primitive ability to reach and grasp. Professionals may be tempted to describe a *clumsy* child as showing minimal signs of brain damage, when what they really mean is that the child's motor co-ordination is immature.

Identifying motor difficulties

It would be unusual for a child coming up to nursery or school age to present marked symptoms of motor difficulty which had not been picked up by the first medical screenings or health visitor checks. However, there are some children with mild symptoms who may hitherto have escaped attention. Teachers may first observe a problem when a child is reluctant to join in games or PE and is markedly less competent than the rest of the group. Clumsiness in large movements will be apparent in hopping, jumping and kicking a ball, walking along a line, stepping between obstacles, accurate throwing and catching, marching to a rhythm, together with riding and balancing toys. Children may have poor 'body awareness' and be unable to name or point to specific parts of themselves. There may be confusions between left and right with no hand preference, usually established by the age of two years.

In fine motor skills a child's clumsiness will be revealed in manipulating buttons, laces and zips, finger painting, threading beads, picking up small objects like matchsticks, using scissors, pegboards and jigsaws, drawing and writing. Drawing and copying shapes or letters requires not only fine eye–hand co-ordination, but also good perceptual skills. The child has first to discriminate the distinctive features of shapes before an attempt can be made to draw them. It is often the case that children with severe co-ordination problems will also have perceptual problems. One complicating factor in both motor and perceptual weaknesses is that children who start out with difficulties usually have fewer opportunities to develop and practise their skills.

In order to help teachers decide whether a child's behaviour is a matter for concern, table 3.3 lists the motor accomplishments of a normal child during the early years. Should a child appear to have passed normal developmental milestones in other areas but show poor fine or gross motor skills, more than a year out of step with expectations for that age, then it would be wise to ask for further

Table 3.3 *Fine and gross motor development in young children*

Age	Gross motor skills	Fine motor skills
6 months	Hold head erect Sits with slight support	Reaches and grasps Shakes rattle
9 months	Stands when held Stepping reaction	Picks up using finger and thumb Passes a toy from one hand to the other
1 year	Walks when led Pulls self up against furniture	Holds a pencil Points with index finger
1½ years	Walks alone well Climbs stairs holding rail or hand Pushes toy pram	Straight scribble using pencil Pincer grip to pick up object like a bead Preference for one hand
2 years	Kicks ball Jumps with two feet together Climbs on furniture	Circular scribble and straight lines Can build a tower of six bricks Pours water from one cup to another
3 years	Stands briefly on one foot Stands and walks on tiptoes Manages stairs one foot per step	Cuts with scissors Copies a circle and line Threads small beads
4 years	Hops on one foot Rides a tricycle Runs fast	Draws a recognisable man with a few features Cuts around and pastes simple shapes Screws large threaded objects together
5 years	Keeps a swing in motion Walks a balance beam Hits nail with hammer	Cuts strip off edge of paper Draws man or house with many features Holds pencil to copy and write over
6 years	Bounces and catches a large ball Skips with alternate feet Hits ball with bat	Prints own name Colours within an outline shape Manages buckles, laces, and buttons
7 years	Rides a bicycle Catches ball in one hand Hangs from a bar bearing own weight	Writes figures 1 to 9 neatly Copies a triangle and diamond Sews using needle

advice. Having first shared any worries with parents, the school nurse, medical officer, PE specialist, or a visiting teacher for the physically handicapped should be able to offer an opinion. Some children brought forward for the first time in school benefit from the help of a physiotherapist or occupational therapist and may require further investigation of their physical problems.

Learning and motor difficulties

Children who have severe motor difficulties, such as those associated with cerebral palsy, may have additional learning obstacles. Motor difficulties often go together with other effects of brain injury, such as epilepsy, hearing or visual impairment, and limited ability to learn. Epilepsy, even of a mild form where the child has 'blank spells' rather than 'fits', interferes with the continuity of the learning process. Such a child may be protected from certain kinds of social contact and experience, there may be side effects from any medication prescribed, whilst the child is quite likely to have problems in concentrating and paying attention over long periods of time.

In order to learn, children not only require intact senses of vision and hearing, but they also have to be capable of attending to important stimuli, making sense of information received, and relating input from different senses to create an orderly whole. In some severe cases, factors causing co-ordination problems also affect the brain's capacity to organise auditory and visual perceptions. Such a child may be distracted by irrelevant information in a busy environment like a normal classroom. There may be impulsive, poorly-controlled reactions to some events and over-exaggerated responses to others. Aggressive or destructive outbursts might be precipitated by seemingly trivial circumstances.

Some learning difficulties arise directly from damage to the brain's functioning; others arise indirectly from effects on the child's experience. As we saw earlier, in chapter 2, the period of sensori-motor exploration in infancy, when the child actively discovers the physical environment, is very important for early language and thinking. There is a close relationship between how we perceive and experience the world, and how language develops to help shape and make sense of our perceptual experiences. For the child with severe motor difficulties, the quality and extent of early experience may be disrupted because the child cannot explore so fully.

There are, then, many reasons to suspect that a child with damage to the central nervous system will have learning difficulties, particularly in language. Both direct and indirect effects can be pin-pointed. In some children we have clear evidence, such as fits, that parts of the brain are not working properly. Effects on the child's learning and behaviour will then depend on which parts of the brain are damaged. For example, the lower parts of the brain, including the cerebellum, are concerned with balance and co-ordination. Injuries to the temporal and frontal lobes of the brain are likely to produce disorders of speech, listening and memory. Some areas of the brain are more specialised than others in language processing, although for many purposes, the brain functions as an organised complex whole. Nevertheless, an injury to the areas of the brain involved in the comprehension and use of linguistic information may result in a child being unable to develop a wide range of language skills.

In a brain-injured child there may be difficulties in discriminating perceptually between the sounds heard in words, even though hearing is good. The child may not recognise that two sounds are the same, or different. The child may be unable, at will, to produce muscle movements in order to articulate the sounds in words. The brain may 'know' what it wants to say, but has an organisational problem in sending the nerve signals to the muscles to make a rhythmical sequence of sounds. The child may have difficulty starting a word, as well as controlling how the sound comes out. In some children, the motor difficulties are focussed specifically upon the vocal organs, so that there are problems moving the tongue around the mouth, in chewing, sucking, swallowing and smiling. The severely brain-injured child may have a wider and more fundamental problem in understanding and using symbols such as gestures, pictures, written symbols, as well as spoken words. This is a much more deep-seated disability affecting the child's ability to think and reason linguistically, which might prevent a child from developing any meaningful communication at all.

Very rarely can such a primary, physical basis for a language disability be identified. We are not often in a position to observe signs of brain damage in any real sense: we hazard a guess from the child's behaviour and development. The picture is complicated because, at the time of birth, the central nervous system is incomplete and changes in development occur in early infancy. So, an infant's brain is *versatile*, and if one part is damaged, some of the functions can be taken over by another part. A young child is less likely to suffer permanent effects of brain injury than is an older person. The nature and effects of an underlying physical difficulty will be modified both by the brain's natural recovery of damaged processes and the child's response to experience and learning opportunity.

We have urged some caution in referring to children as being 'brain damaged', when we really mean that they are clumsy and poorly co-ordinated, with signs of immaturity in concentration and self-control. If there are no clear signs of brain damage, such as epilepsy, the cause cannot be identified unequivocally and we are really only describing a pattern of behaviour which may, or may not, be due to neurological damage. The safest approach is to stick closely to what the child can and cannot do, perhaps using a checklist of age-appropriate behaviours (see table 3.3) as a framework for assessment.

Spina bifida

Not all children with damage to the central nervous system have learning difficulties. Children with spina bifida are born with a defect of the spinal column in which the arches of one or more of the spinal vertebrae have failed to fuse together, exposing the nerves and their protective sheathing. The term 'spina bifida' embraces a group of defects, the physical consequences of which depend upon how high up the spinal column the lesion occurs and the amount of damage incurred to the spinal cord and its surrounding membranes. In less severe forms the vertebral arches do not fuse, but the cord and its membranes may be normal. There may be no external evidence of the defect, apart from a slight swelling or dimple in the skin, and function is hardly affected. In more severe cases some of the spinal cord tissue protrudes into a sac-like cyst filled with cerebro-spinal fluid, and the cord itself is abnormal. The result is a permanent neurological defect leading to incontinence, paralysis of the legs and perceptuo-motor difficulties. Hydrocephalus, or excess fluid within the brain, is a complication of spina bifida which can cause further damage to the central nervous system. As we have said, many children with spina bifida have normal learning abilities and participate, with the appropriate practical help to overcome specific problems, such as mobility, in ordinary mainstream schools (Anderson and Spain, 1977).

It is sometimes said that some spina bifida children show the 'Cocktail Party Syndrome'. What is meant by this is that a child has a good fluency of expressive language and can chatter about a wide range of topics. The child uses a wealth of vocabulary and shows excellent control of complex grammatical structures. Words and phrases are picked up quickly and used readily, giving an impression of quick thinking and clear understanding. However, the child may not have such good understanding as people are led to believe. Words may be used with little meaning behind them. The child may have limited reasoning skills and be unable to keep what is said relevant to the conversation context. The 'Cocktail Party Syndrome' is so named because of an inability to keep talk relevant and meaningful, with a tendency to use language superficially and without true comprehension. It arises, primarily, because of the problems children have when they are limited in their mobility, in tying language to direct experience.

Cleft palate

A cleft palate occurs when tissues which should have grown in towards each other to form the roof of the mouth fail to do so. Sometimes this occurs together with a split in the upper lip, often referred to as a 'hare lip'. These conditions have a large genetic component and may run in families. They may occur in conjunction with other defects such as a visual impairment. The palate and lip tissues are normally joined by the third month of pregnancy, but in approximately 1 per 1000 births this fusion has not occurred, although the precise breakdown in the mechanisms involved is unclear. A child needs a whole palate and lips in order to have a normal appearance, to eat properly, and to speak. Surgical corrections are usually performed within the first year of life.

What kind of speech problems are associated with cleft palate? Depending on the severity of the cleft and the success of any repairs attempted, the child may have some difficulty in articulating speech sounds involving the lips and palate. Children born with a cleft palate are often unable to breathe properly through the mouth and it may take a long time to regulate correct patterns of airflow essential for speech. If air is lost through the nose, many sounds, such as the fricative 'f' or 's', will lose their clarity and be pronounced nasally. In fact, other kinds of palatal problems can produce similar effects on speech. If there is a weakness in muscular control of the soft palate, the child may have difficulty in producing some of the sound contrasts and have a very nasal voice quality. Other children are quick to seize upon any difference in appearance or voice such physical abnormalities cause and there are almost always additional psychological consequences.

Children with cleft palate may show delays in other areas of language, such as using and understanding vocabulary and complex syntax. The most likely explanation for this lies in the very high risk cleft palate brings of fluctuating hearing loss. Cleft palate children tend to suffer a lot of colds and flu because mouth breathing promotes infection. We have already discussed the mechanism by which such infections pass into the middle ear. In cleft palate children, because of the weakness in the palate muscles which operate the eustachian tube, the middle ear may be poorly ventilated. Because of these factors conductive hearing loss affects up to 90 per cent of children with cleft palate (Northern and Downs, 1978). It is realistic to consider any child with a physical abnormality of the ear, nose or throat, as being at risk of middle ear disease and fluctuating hearing loss. What this means is that such children are likely to show the wide range of speech and language difficulties which are commonly associated with a mild hearing loss.

LIMITED ABILITY

We cannot assume that every child is blessed with a similar ability to learn. Children respond differently to the learning opportunities they have and will vary, not only in the quickness with which they pick up a new skill, but also in their style of approaching a learning task. These differences may be obvious in babyhood. For example, a child of one of the authors spent many months shuffling along on her bottom and hesitantly holding onto furniture, before finally setting out independently to walk a few steps. This was a kind of gradual building up of confidence and skill, literally 'step by step'. In the same family a later baby decided confidently to shift from sitting to walking overnight, without a practice stage. These contrasting styles of learning, one gradual and methodical, the other rapid but high risk, characterise each child's behaviour in many aspects of their lives to date.

One familiar way of determining whether a child has a learning difficulty is to administer some kind of intelligence test. Many educational psychologists now regard this as a relatively unimportant aspect of their work, although by tradition, when a referral is made to a school psychologist, it might be expected that the child will be asked to complete an IQ test. The Wechsler Intelligence Scale for Children – Revised is, perhaps, the IQ test most used with school-aged children in the United Kingdom. This has two parts – a series of question-and-answer type problems which give a measure of verbal abilities; and a performance scale of tasks which are less dependent on language for their completion. On the verbal scale a child might be asked general knowledge questions, arithmetic problems, or questions designed to elicit the child's knowledge of simple concepts. The verbal items demand a range of skills from the child, including memory for facts, thinking, reasoning, and ability to express ideas coherently in speech. Some of the individual differences revealed by giving this test will reflect the child's social experience together with what has been learnt in school. The non-verbal, or performance, scale consists of a range of picture, block, and puzzle tasks, which the child has to assemble, sequence or manipulate in some way. These tests rely mainly on good fine motor co-ordination, vision, and perceptual skills, and to a lesser degree on language. The end product of such an assessment is a verbal IQ and a performance IQ, with a full scale IQ score summarising the whole. A list of the WISC–R subtests, and what they reveal, is given in table 3.4.

IQ tests such as the WISC–R have, at their core, an assumption that learning ability is distributed evenly across the child population. A normal statistical distribution assumes that half of the population fall below, and half above, a theoretical average point. At one end of the spectrum there will be a number of 'gifted', academically capable children who are quick to learn. These are counterbalanced, at the other end of the spectrum, by a few children who experience serious difficulties in learning. This latter group may have good vision and hearing, with no reason to suspect that brain damage or adverse environmental factors have impaired the child's intelligence. On the other hand there may be a number of children at this lower end of the spectrum who do have a known handicapping condition, together with a wide range of obstacles to learning, such as epilepsy, visual loss, and motor disability. Children described as 'mentally-handicapped' may have been so classified on the basis of an IQ test. Whilst an effort is sometimes made to differentiate learning disability from the effects of mental retardation, sensory defects, and social or emotional factors, in practice, the learning problems of individual children are usually complex and interlinked. It would, for example, be extremely difficult to separate the effects of a child's feelings of school failure from the effects of the learning difficulty itself. In fact, one major criticism of traditional IQ tests is that, whilst they may give a general indication of a child's overall ability in relation to other children (the IQ score), very little is gleaned about the individual child's functional mastery of important learning skills across the educational curriculum. A separate, skill-related assessment procedure would be necessary to reveal this kind of information about a child.

What kind of features appear to characterise children who are learning-disabled? It may be that the first noticeable characteristics are that a child is late to reach developmental milestones, such as talking, sitting or walking, in comparison with other children of the same age. A range of new skills may be grasped only slowly, whilst a pattern of behaviour may have to be repeated over and again before it can safely said to have been added to the child's repertoire. In school the child may stand out as being 'limited' in several respects. There may be immaturity in social independence skills, in taking responsibility for personal hygiene and avoiding danger, together with a pattern of emotional behaviour, such as inability to take turns or wait, tantrums and upsets typical of a younger age range. The child's strategies for learning, in terms of attention-span, distractibility and ability to work without adult help, are also revealing. So

Table 3.4 *Subtests of the Wechsler Intelligence Scale for Children – Revised*

Verbal Scale		Performance Scale	
Information	(general knowledge questions, e.g. number of things in a dozen)	Picture completion	(visual awareness, e.g. spotting missing details such as the spokes in an umbrella)
Comprehension	(social reasoning, e.g. why we have policemen, car number plates)	Picture arrangement	(sequencing, e.g. putting a series of pictures into the correct order to tell a sensible story)
Arithmetic	(verbal arithmetic, e.g. basic operations including simple money sums)	Block design	(visuo-perceptual skills, e.g. matching blocks to a picture template)
Similarities	(verbal concepts, e.g. how two objects such as a piano and a guitar are alike)	Object assembly	(re-constituting jigsaws of objects such as a car)
Vocabulary	(expressive skills, e.g. the meaning of a word like 'mantis')	Coding	(a series of numbers or signs has to be written into a given code)
Digit span	(short-term memory for a series of numbers)	Mazes	(planning a pencil route through a maze to reach a goal)

too, the kind of general features identified by the WISC profile, such as reasoning ability, memory for facts, social awareness, persistence at a mechanical task, range of vocabulary and concepts, and ability to plan and organise a task, all indicate that a child is less well prepared for learning than the majority of the peer group. The basic rudiments of reading, writing, and numerical skills, may be difficult to acquire, without a great deal of individual help and small, finely-graded learning steps. In fact, there is a fairly extensive literature on children with global learning difficulties (see, for example, Devereux, 1981). In this section we shall be concentrating on two major aspects: the nature of the language problems experienced by slow-learning children, and the effects of learning handicaps on the behaviour of adult caretakers.

Language and the slow learner

It has been said that the particular difficulties experienced by slow-learning children in language create 'an almost insurmountable barrier to cognitive development and educational progress' (Graham, 1980, page 69). According to this view it is the child's problems in using language which are at the root of the child's learning difficulty. For example, slowness in building up a store of vocabulary inevitably means that the child is slower in organising and shaping perceptions and experience. Similarly, a less sophisticated control of the complexities of sentence structure may lead to a more limited ability to relate one concept to another, or to make categories and generalisations. We presume, too, that the amount of 'inner language' the child has available for manipulating concepts and dealing with events in the abstract, is dependent on prior developments in the child's spoken communication and understanding. This is essentially the Soviet position on language and thinking, discussed in chapter 2. Language mediates the child's experience and provides the basic structure for thinking. The increasing intellectual demands made upon children as they move through the school system seem to point towards a greater dependence on abstract modes of thought. In order to develop hypothetical thinking, whereby the child can infer relationships, situations, and events beyond the 'here and now', the child has to have a sophisticated grasp of language.

An alternative view is that the child discovers important objects and their relationships in the environment, and then seeks ways to express these concepts in language. This is essentially the Piagetian view, that language merely reflects and expresses what the child has already discovered through exploration and play.

What kind of cognitive restraints might limit the child's early discovery of the world? For the slow learning child we might include poor attention span and an inability to select important information. The child might have a limited memory for sequences of events, together with problems in identifying and relating one feature to another. An underlying difficulty may be one of representing an experience away from the original situation, with a need for a great deal of repetition before experience is eventually absorbed. To give a more specific example, if a child is only capable of holding two items of information in short-term memory when asked to remember a series of everyday, familiar objects, one might predict a difficulty in using sentence structures with more than two or three elements of meaning. The child's limited capacity to hold information in brief store constrains the language rules and processes that can be used.

A compromise view is that language is not really a *product* of learning, but a *process* of development. Language disabilities are not so much precursors, or consequences, of the child's general ability to learn as a part of the nexus of behaviour to which the term 'learning disability' is applied. As such, the focus of interest moves away from children and their deficits, towards factors outside the child, in the learning context. One psychologist who has recognised the importance of the conditions in which learning takes place is Gagné (1977). A lot of what Gagné has to say about situations surrounding learning fits in well with the model of language development adopted in this book and accounts for many of the learning problems experienced by children of limited abilities.

Gagné's theory begins with an identification of the broad categories of skill which children acquire during development. These include using symbols in speech, intellectual activities such as classifying and analysing objects, and literacy skills. He also highlights the giving of information to others, or the conveying of ideas. Skills to manage learning are also important, such as attention, memory, and problem-solving strategies. Gagné then suggests that, whereas the child's 'genetic stock' cannot be altered, factors that influence learning are largely determined by events in the environment. In other words, children come into the world with differing sets of attributes, capacities and potentials, but it is the events which children live through at home, in school, and in other social environments, which influence what children can become. For each area of skill identified, Gagné is able to define what it is that the child brings to the learning task, and how conditions affect what is learned.

Gagné gives the example of a child learning concepts such as the object qualities of red, circular, and smooth. At first, the child may make the simple tactile discrimination that an object is 'smooth' or 'not smooth'. However, the child can be guided or 'cued' into making the discrimination by the introduction of the word 'smooth'. This aside, concepts will be learnt much more quickly if the child is able to discover the object quality by having several instances in which to experience smoothness, when other object characteristics, such as size or weight, are varied. Important conditions for learning are that the child understands the purpose of the exercise; the concept is self-generated, rather than being handed over by the teacher as information to be accepted; the learning involves direct experience of a range of exploratory situations where it is the child who has to make decisions; and the teacher provides feedback and encouragement. Not all concepts need to be learned by direct interaction, but it is the teacher's job to work out the child's current level of understanding and to plan appropriate step-by-step experiences in order to move the child on from stage to stage. In a sense, these principles apply whatever the intellectual skills of the child. In chapter 5, we shall be seeing the practical implications of Gagné's approach in the classroom.

Adult–child interactions with learning-disabled children

One important area of research on the influence of the learning context concerns the nature of interactions between adults and children who are perceived as being 'handicapped'. We know that the expectations which adults hold of children's potential has a significant impact on their achievements. Children with known handicapping conditions, such as a severe hearing-impairment, may become victims of the labels which are attached to them. If it is widely believed that such a group of children are bound to make poor educational progress, then these beliefs may be self-fulfilling. Unwittingly, the spontaneous behaviour of adults may change towards less nurturing styles of interaction, if it is known before-hand that the child has a learning difficulty.

Down's syndrome children have often been selected for study because of their distinctive physical appearance. Not all Down's children have severe learning difficulties, although many show developmental delay in acquiring a range of skills, particularly in language. Adults may expect a Down's child to be immature, to need greater help and protection, and to show less understanding than normal. One question which has been asked is whether, when comparisons are made with normal children, adults make the same demands on Down's children and provide the same degree of language interaction. That question is perhaps more straightforward to answer than the knotty problem of whether it is the child, or the adult, who influences the other's behaviour most of all. A summary of this area of research has been given by Mitchell (1976).

The pooled findings of this research suggest that Down's children tend to be talked to frequently, but with the use of shorter, simpler, and more incomplete sentences than normal. Measures of language complexity, such as tense forms, pronouns, and conjunctions, show that adults tend to use less complex language with the Down's group. There is a greater tendency to ask questions, particularly of the kind where the adult already knows the answer. The adult more frequently commands, controls, and prohibits the child and gives more physical prompts. Of course, the context in which learning takes place can be changed. The quality of adult interactions with learning-disabled children can be improved by suggesting more productive strategies for talking, playing, and learning together. This is precisely the emphasis we have given to remedial intervention in chapter 5. Accepting that the locus of the problem does not always lie within the child paves the way for modifying aspects of the learning setting, through which a child, whatever the learning difficulties, is helped towards more effective learning.

PSYCHOLOGICAL FACTORS

Children's social and emotional well-being is intimately related to the normal development of communication skills. Two aspects are considered here, though it is difficult to separate them entirely. On the one hand, a child's problems in using and developing language may be felt to have an emotional basis. In the absence of any underlying sensory, physical or intellectual disability, emotional disturbance may play a large part. Elective mutism can be considered in these terms, when children select the circumstances in which they feel confident enough to communicate. Where a child presents a more severe psychiatric disturbance, such as infantile autism, there may well be hidden neurological or perceptual deficits which contribute to the child's difficulties, although the precise mechanisms are not fully understood.

On the other hand, it is well known that children who experience language difficulties also tend to develop educational and social problems as a consequence. Parents often describe the florid temper tantrums of children, which are perhaps the result of the sheer frustration of being unable to communicate wishes and needs effectively. Parents who are unable to explain to children why they must take turns, give a toy back, return home early from a friend's or avoid potential hazards such as road traffic, may resort to physical controls and risk a temper outburst instead. So relationships may become fraught and emotionally charged as a result of communication difficulties.

Elective mutism

Some children are silent except with a small group of familiar people and in familiar surroundings. It is often observed that when children start nursery or find themselves in a strange environment, such as a hospital waiting room, they will not talk, or will only do so in a whisper. This is a normal reaction which reflects a temporary feeling of anxiety. Such children will generally chatter freely on home territory where they feel more comfortable. However, there are a few children who remain silent for periods from one month up to several years, in situations to which children usually become accustomed fairly quickly. Prolonged difficulty in prompting a child to talk in contexts like the classroom, is referred to as elective mutism.

Mutism is slightly more common in girls than boys, unlike many kinds of speech and language difficulty. There is no known physical or intellectual basis for it and it is fairly rare, perhaps affecting less than 1 child in a 1000 (Fundudis, Kolvin, and Garside, 1979). Occasionally, it occurs in more than one child from the same family and in twins. Mutism is often first noticed on entry to primary school but has been reported at secondary transfer. If one tried to find similarities between electively mute children or their families, few common traits would be identified. Some children have histories of speech defects, or excessive shyness, whilst others have parents who are socially isolated or have received psychiatric treatment. But there are rather more differences than factors in common.

Jessica, a child referred to one of the authors at the age of eight and a half years, had not spoken to anyone in school since the time she arrived, when five years old. She was a withdrawing, timid and fearful girl, who had no friends in school and avoided any social contact. Other aspects of her behaviour suggested tense, neurotic traits, such as her obsession with tidiness and being neat and clean. Jessica's mother, too, was a solitary figure who preferred to stay indoors rather than meet people. The family lived at the top of a high-rise block of flats which meant that they did not meet their neighbours easily. The mother would bring Jessica right to the classroom door just after the school day had started. Teachers had a strong sense of the child being overprotected at home.

In this kind of situation, where a child appears to be so unresponsive in school, teachers themselves feel distressed. They may have tried all the strategies they know of, and which have worked with other shy children, in prompting them to talk. Repeated failure to establish contact with a child may make a teacher feel inadequate, guilty, or angry. Other school staff may attempt to manoeuvre a child into speaking, which just seems to make the impasse harder to escape from. The first thing to establish is whether the child talks in other situations and whether progress is being made in schoolwork. In Jessica's case she did talk a great deal to her family, with no apparent problems in speech pronunciation, vocabulary, or sentence structure. She appeared to understand instructions in class, produced work at an appropriate level, and enjoyed reading to herself. Teachers may be able to reassure themselves, on some counts, that all is not lost when a child chooses to be silent with them, and the eventual outcome for elective mutes is usually positive.

Jessica's mutism could be seen as part of a family problem in relating adequately to the social stresses of the outside world. The school sought help from its visiting educational psychologist, who subsequently involved a family social worker. Ways were suggested to the family for helping them negotiate by degrees some of their day-to-day social stress points. Jessica herself was helped by spending some time every week with a play therapist who introduced her to a small group of children with whom she felt safe and secure. A potential problem was avoided with her younger sister, who was approaching school age, by the infant teacher visiting the family at home and introducing materials and play activities. The teacher became part of the context in which the child spoke. The gradual aim of any strategy to help an elective mute is to increase the range of settings in which the child speaks. Having become used to talking whilst the infant teacher was present, it was easier for Jessica's sister to speak at school. Generally, teachers are advised not to highlight the problems by demanding verbal contributions; to encourage a child to work in a small group with familiar, non-threatening children; to reward with praise or a favoured activity when the child does begin to speak; and to remember that not speaking does not always mean a child is not learning. (For further discussion, see Kratochwill, 1981.)

Stuttering

The terms 'stuttering' or 'stammering' usually refer to disturbances in the fluency of speech. In some instances an individual might be blocked from making any initial sound and struggles to release the air-flow. In other cases a part or whole of a word is prolonged or repeated, as in 'What t-t-t-time is it, pl-pl-please?' Occasionally, extra words are introduced such as 'erm', whilst other words might be left unfinished. Some stutterers are aware of the kinds of sounds which cause them problems and go to great lengths to avoid them by choosing round about ways of describing what they mean. Other children who stutter may have an additional problem in word-finding, the ability to retrieve from memory a specific word needed to express an idea. Rutherford (1977) suggests that 35–50 per cent of young stutterers also have word-finding problems. Characteristic features of most stutterers are an awkward hesitancy of speech rhythm, and irregular patterns of stress and breathing. The problem is not restricted so much to sounds, as to the whole organisation of speech production.

Why do people stutter? All sorts of reasons have been put forward, ranging from damage to the areas of the brain controlling speech timing, to inherited factors. We must be careful not to confuse stuttering with the usual hesitancy in speech found in young children. Pauses, repetition and non-fluency are normal features of speech, especially when a situation is exciting or unfamiliar. The problem of stuttering is certainly intensified by the social context. Most explanations of stuttering include a psychological component, with anxiety and embarrassment playing a major role. Fear of not being able to produce a word or sentence correctly, perhaps at the point at which a child is trying to master a more complex syntax pattern, undoubtedly makes the stuttering worse. Advice about children who stutter should always be sought from a speech therapist. There are several approaches which can help. Counselling, relaxation programmes, and techniques such as delaying auditory feedback to the speaker using headphones and tape-recorder all claim success.

Twins

There are some unexpected kinds of language difficulty in which psychological factors play a part, such as the speech delay often found in twins. Families where there are multiple births provide less parent–child interaction than is possible with single births. Twins spend a lot of time in each other's company and may develop a secret language which can only be understood by the co-twin. It is inevitable that much less time is spent communicating with older children, and children of the same age may be less stimulating than older siblings or adults. In consequence it is often found that twins have more limited vocabularies and less sophisticated sentence structure, and may be less competent in language tasks at school than peers. (For a summary of twin research, see Mittler, 1971.)

'Deaf' environment

One of the important influences on the development of children's language which we have already highlighted, is the quality of a mother's speech to her child. We must be careful not to equate social class differences with verbal deprivation. Evidence already cited also suggests that children who are badly neglected in the early years may eventually overcome the developmental problems which result from extreme social isolation. However, there is one unusual family situation which may be thought to have an unavoidable effect on otherwise normal offspring: hearing children of deaf parents.

What effects are there on speech and language growth, when children are exposed to atypical speech patterns and a parental language of sign? We know that deaf adults may pronounce words in a way which is unintelligible to strangers. Some sounds may be distorted, others omitted, whilst speech rhythms may become slow and flat. Many deaf adults continue to have serious problems in using the complex structures of English grammar. This is not to say, of course, that communication between deaf people is not rich and subtle. Using signs, deaf parents would be able to communicate a sophisticated range of vocabulary and concepts to their hearing children. But how do these children fare in relation to hearing children, for example, upon entry to school?

In the few studies that have been carried out in this area (Schiff and Ventry, 1976) most children seem to learn two systems of communication: one with hearing people and one with those who are deaf. With the latter at home, or in a club for deaf people, the child may use an elaborate range of gestures and signs, together with speech rhythms and intonation patterns resembling 'deaf' speech. In contacts with the hearing world the same child may develop a separate language system of normal speech sounds and vocabulary, following a normal sequence in acquiring the stages of grammar. It is quite likely, however, since the amount of contact with hearing adults will be less frequent, that the child's 'hearing' system of language will be delayed in comparison with similar-aged children in a typical family. An important influence on this will be the range of contacts the child has with hearing adults and children, such as relatives, neighbours, at playgroup, or nursery. It would be very rare for a child not to have any contact at all with 'hearing' communication, if only through the television or radio.

Depending, then, on the quality and frequency of the different speech environments, presence of hearing siblings, and how well the parents themselves communicate, children of deaf parents are quite likely to need additional help. The articulation patterns, stress, and rhythms of 'deaf' speech may persist in the child's communication in 'hearing' settings and the child may be unintelligible to strangers. There may be problems in understanding and using complex sentence structures and a limited vocabulary. Some of the errors, omissions, and confusions reported in the speech and grammar of deaf individuals may be reflected in the child who hears these deviant patterns at home. Approximately half of the hearing children of deaf parents in Schiff and Ventry's (1976) study had communication problems. In every instance, the children's speech was better than the parent's own. Six of the 52 children reported on turned out to have undiagnosed hearing losses requiring hearing aids. Parents had usually been told whether their child was 'hearing' or 'deaf' in babyhood and did not suspect otherwise.

Teachers and professionals who come into contact with this unusual group of children should be aware that some hearing losses are progressive and may only come to light later on in childhood. Deaf parents who see their child responding to sounds may find it hard to accept that their child does have a hearing disability after all. On a wider note, deaf adults as a group often feel very isolated and threatened in relation to a hearing society in which they find participation difficult. Hearing children may discover some conflicting social attitudes as they leave the family.

Emotional trauma and 'deprivation'

Every so often national newspapers and television reports draw public attention to the plight of children who have been subject to abuse and neglect. In some instances children are locked away in back bedrooms, starved of food and physically battered. Some unfortunate children are discovered too late and whilst the parents may be brought to justice, nothing can assuage the suffering inflicted. Some children survive periods of early neglect and social isolation. The evidence we reviewed in chapters 1 and 2 suggests that the satisfactory all-round development of children depends on a nurturing and fulfilling family environment. Badly neglected children fail to thrive in their physical growth; they may have a very restricted range of experiences from which to learn; they may be scarred emotionally, with deep feelings of insecurity and anxiety.

Language is perhaps the area of development most likely to show severe delays when the normal processes of social interaction have been denied. Fortunately, as Skuse (1984) suggests, children are very robust creatures. Children removed from socially depriving situations into families which provide care and love often overcome the ill effects of early neglect. Rapid recovery in all areas of development, including language, can be anticipated once social conditions are put right.

There are some social environments which are less than good, without necessarily being neglectful. Families beset with problems, such as the death of a child, divorce, a very handicapped sibling, unemployment, an adult seriously ill in hospital, or poor living conditions, may find it impossible to give consistent care and attention to all its members. Some families cope very well with emotional crises, others disintegrate. Individual children also react differently. A child whose mother dies may show little reaction. Another child temporarily separated from the family because of a hospital operation may react by withdrawal and a period of mutism.

Autism

There will be few people whose interest has not been captured by autistic children. These children are often described mysteriously as 'beautiful yet inaccessible', given to treating other people like objects, never smiling or responding, locked in a private world. We have been careful to avoid the stereotyping inherent in medical labels. Instead, we have focussed on the factors which seem to characterise an individual's behaviour. This approach is appropriate to the children often grouped under the syndrome of autism. Indeed, only a minute proportion of autistic children display all of the traits which are thought to be characteristic (or 'classic'). What are the behavioural features which mark these children so distinctively?

The term 'autism' was applied originally because of the disturbed nature of the child's social interactions with others, so particularly distressing to parents. As babies, they may be placid and undemanding, or the opposite extreme: restless and implacable, with screaming, head-banging and disturbed sleep. Some autistic babies resist cuddling and do not reach out to be picked up. There may be little interest in adults or their voices, and limited curiosity in the environment. It is around the age of three years that parents often realise something is badly wrong. The child may panic at the slightest change in routine, such as walking a new route to the shops, or if someone sits in a different place at the table. Despite the lack of attachment to people, there may be obsessions such as collecting keys, bottles, or stones. Toys may be played with repetitively by spinning, twisting or turning, rather than imaginatively. Ritual behaviour such as hand-flapping or rocking may be observed. Lack of fear of traffic, heights or water, may be combined with an irrational terror of harmless objects. Autistic children may look through people rather than at them. They may pay no attention to intense sounds, but be fascinated by the touch or smell of an object. A few children show narrow, special abilities, such as memorising all the Derby winners; whilst there are severe difficulties in other areas of learning.

There have been many theories about the cause of autism. Originally, it was thought that the disturbance was emotional and bound up in a cold mother–child relationship. The more recent view (Wing, 1976) is that autism results from an inability to make sense of incoming information. The fact that many autistic children later develop epilepsy suggests that brain damage may be a root cause (Deykin and MacMahon, 1979). This does not explain why most brain-damaged children do not show symptoms of autism. It appears likely that the central disturbance is linked to language, if only because the autistic children who do achieve any degree of social adjustment are those who acquire some useful communication skills. However, whilst language training with autistic children appears to hold the key to progress, there are no guarantees attached to any one particular teaching method (Rutter, 1980).

The language disorders of autistic children are part of much broader cognitive difficulties involving ordering, abstracting, and learning from experience. For example, panic reactions to change may stem from an inability to appreciate the factors which do remain similar from one situation to the next. Rooms are still familiar to most people even though the furniture is moved around, because we recognise and abstract the essential features. In autism, all forms of symbolic function may be affected, including gesturing, imaginative playing, imitating sounds, using and comprehending speech, as well as reading and writing. One feature which demonstrates the child's poor understanding of language is echolalia. Whole phrases heard previously may be repeated in totally inappropriate contexts. Some autistic children have difficulty with personal pronouns in their speech, perhaps reversing 'I' and 'you'. A child might say 'You go home' when he clearly means himself. This could be a normal developmental confusion shown by many two-year-olds, which has simply persisted. However, the earlier view of autism took pronoun reversals to be symptoms of a lack of identity, whereby the self is not distinguished from others.

The majority of autistic children show language which is both immature and deviant. The child might be arrested at an early stage of, say, three-element grammatical structures. There may never be an occasion on which sentences are produced spontaneously for social purposes, to greet, express feelings, or ask for something. Prompts may have to be given before the child responds at all. Inevitably, all kinds of symbols hold no meaning. Attention has been drawn to the social aloofness and emotional indifference which autistic children show towards people. However, it seems likely that the primary problem of autism is a cognitive one, perhaps due to brain damage, affecting the use and understanding of language in all its forms.

Emotional consequences of language problems

> *On the first occasion that the authors visited David's family, he had to be prised off the top of a dining room cabinet. The house bore the scars of David's frequent misdemeanours and temper outbursts. He had stripped paper off the walls, cut holes in the carpet and broken most of the glass panels in the doors. David had two ordinary brothers and sisters, although he himself experienced severe expressive communication difficulties. He could not make himself understood and his parents lost patience trying to make him understand. David could not be taken anywhere because his mother was afraid he would throw a tantrum. Few children came to the house to play. As time went on and David reached four, his parents became increasingly angry at his slowness in speaking. Mother, particularly, resorted to shouting and punishing David by smacking. That way he clearly comprehended that he had done something amiss. However, relationships in the family became very heavily charged. The parents were unable to see anything good about David and he was never praised. His mother had once said that if David had been a dog, they would have had him 'put down'. He continued to destroy furniture and toys until the point at which he was able to make himself clearly understood. Only then did some of the frustrations and the need for physical controls begin to lessen. Eventually David attended a school where he could have daily speech therapy help and his behaviour slowly improved.*

In our experience children who have problems in communicating are highly likely to be affected in their behaviour and emotional development as well. Since language is the medium through which children achieve and sustain social contact with peers and adults, it is not surprising that language difficulties disturb social interaction. Children may become so distressed at their own inability to reach others through speech that they avoid contact altogether and withdraw into themselves. Alternatively, they release their frustration by hitting out, and draw attention to themselves by upsetting others. In the past such children may have achieved their aim by screaming, and this pattern of demanding behaviour can persist. When a child has limited language many of the activities enjoyed by other children of the same age, either at play or in school, are not so rewarding. Children who cannot join in at the same level as peers may become clinging, disruptive, or simply feel badly about themselves.

Children with poor language often earn themselves reputations in school for being distractible, unable to settle to a task, restless, and lacking in concentration. When things go wrong there may be intense upsets. The smallest change in routine may produce tears.

The child may be unable to anticipate a likely sequence of events, to wait or take turns, whilst sharing requires an ability to see another's point of view, rather than one's own. All of these aspects might typify the child who is felt to be emotionally immature. As the child acquires language, behaviour also improves. (For a summary of the research evidence, see Fundudis, Kolvin, and Garside, 1979.)

SPECIFIC LANGUAGE DIFFICULTIES

There are some children with good vision and hearing, who show no signs of any underlying physical or neurological problem and who may have been shown to have normal intelligence, but who still present language problems. If every other possible factor has been excluded and the child's language is slow or different in some way, compared with normal, we may have to accept that there is a disability specific to the child's learning of language. We are often not in a position to say why or how this arises. Some people will speculate and say that there is damage to the areas of the brain which deal with the processes of speech and language. But that is often pure guess work. All we can do, in most instances, is to describe the areas of language affected and compare a child's development in a specific area, such as speech sounds, with the skills normally acquired by children as they mature. In one sense, terms like 'aphasic' are applied to children with severe difficulties in using and understanding language, when every other explanation, such as deafness, has been ruled out.

Sound articulation

If teachers are asked which group of children are usually dealt with by a speech therapist, many would say children who cannot pronounce sounds clearly. Of course, all children start out by pronouncing words with some sounds missing or changed around. Between the ages of 1 and 3, when rapid developments occur in a wide range of language skills, children begin to pay attention to the important sound contrasts in words and to work out the rules which operate in the adult system. It is quite normal for children to make sound confusions, to reduce the cluster of sounds in a longer word and to substitute one sound for another. The stages through which most children pass as they acquire the sound system of the language, are set out in chapter 2. It was pointed out that there are some sound sequences in words like 'statistics' or 'sixth', which pose problems of pronunciation until the age of nine or ten years.

Bearing in mind the *expected* immaturity in children's pronunciation at a given age, we can assess the degree to which an individual's pronunciation problems cause difficulties in understanding what the child is trying to say. The child may be using a wide range of vocabulary and sentence structures. We may have ruled out any possibility of hearing loss, physical abnormality such as cleft palate, or any underlying motor difficulty affecting muscle co-ordination. The child may have good intelligence, and have lived in an ordinary speech environment. Yet sounds are articulated in such a way that few can understand the child's speech. The difficulties may, at one end of the scale, be fairly mild.

> *Lizzie at four years was unable to pronounce any consonant clusters, such as 'br', 'qu', 'pl', 'gr', or 'pr', which are produced at the front of the mouth using the lips, palate and tongue. In fact, each one of these consonant blends requires a complex sequence of articulatory movements, which can be specified in some detail. Lizzie's general tendency was to simplify the words by substituting sounds requiring fewer movements, so that 'bread' became 'jed', 'quick' became 'shick', 'plum' became 'clum', 'grape' became 'jape', and 'pram' was pronounced 'sham'. Fortunately, these substitutions affected only a narrow range of sounds and, using the sentence context, people could make out what was being said. This holds true for many children whose articulation problem is restricted to a single sound, such as a weak 'r' or lisped 's'.*

Less fortunate are those children whose articulation is affected across a wide range of sound contrasts. Where many sounds appear to be misarticulated a child may be completely unintelligible to others. We usually suspect a difficulty in identifying the important segments of sounds in the speech rhythms being used around the child. A weakness in auditory perception may require a special programme of training to identify the contrasts the child is having problems with and then to provide opportunities for practising these sounds. This is, of course, an important province (although by no means the only one) of the speech therapist. Any teacher who is worried about a child's articulation should seek a speech therapist's advice.

Sentence structure

Some children's language difficulties arise specifically in the area of syntax: the rules which determine how words are sequenced to produce meaning. Grammar can be thought of as the organising principles of language. It accounts for the phrase, clause, and sentence patterns which children eventually master as they mature. In chapter 2 we described the stages which children move through as they use sentence structures of increasing complexity. Most children are able to use very sophisticated sentence patterns by the time they enter school. However, a few children with apparently good hearing, vision, and motor skills, and with no signs of any intellectual disability or brain damage, may show particular problems in grammar. Children may have clearly articulated sounds and a wide range of vocabulary at their disposal. There may be good understanding of things said to the child. But efforts to put words together to express an idea seem to fail.

Examples of deviant sentence patterns

Metal no car fire and some walking monsters made in metal. Got sticker stamps on their feet, to stand their up.
Mummy ring the phone up. Mummy says she I'm ring the phone. Andrew just starts shout and he do and Trixie will bark.
Her is going putting get ready to school.
'Cos I got my tissue in my pocket blow.
Can't me find a pencil.
He got be finish, colour him feets.
A berries comed off.
He has a braking arm. The other day six ago I have a braking and my dad rushed me to hospital.
Cat jumped on the tree. He go to garage, get ladder.
Not Carmen be well.

There are two, distinctly different, kinds of problem which can be identified. Firstly, the child may be stuck at a very immature stage of syntax. For example, a child of six or seven years using structures like 'Where my Mummy gone?', or 'That my drink', which are typical of stage III or IV will be seriously held back in school because of the limitations in expressive powers. This kind of problem we have called a 'language delay'. The second kind of difficulty arises when the child's use of grammar is not only delayed, but also deviant. In other words, the child produces sentence patterns which are not found in the normal stages of development. A selection of deviant sentence structures, from recorded conversations with children, is given above. These examples show obvious confusions in word order, how words are modified in their use with each other, in plurals, verb forms, and appropriate use of pronouns, adjectives, adverbs, prepositions and conjunctions. Phrase and clause patterns are controlled by a different set of rules from normal and there may be many inconsistencies in the child's efforts to create language sequences.

Why should a child have such problems in learning and using sentence structures? One possibility is that the child has a very poor memory for auditory information and rhythms. There are some very simple tests of auditory memory, such as Digit Span on the WISC. The child is asked to recall a series of numbers read out in sequence at one digit per second. Children with speech and language difficulties may be very poor at this kind of test. They may only be able to recall two or three numbers in correct sequence. It is possible, of course, that skill in using language itself develops auditory sequencing ability. However, it seems feasible that the power to remember a long sequence of verbal information will be important in using complex sentence structures. Presumably, a child who can only manage to retain two or three items in short-term memory will not be able to use or understand sentence structures where the meaning is spread across a much greater span of information. Perhaps the problem lies not so much in recalling auditory information in serial form as in reproducing it in an organised rhythmical sequence. This inability to store and organise verbal information may be the root cause of many language disorders. It may be that the child can only produce simple sentence structures, compatible with stages II or III, whilst maintaining other aspects of language: clear articulation, good rhythm, appropriate vocabulary, intonation, and fluency. When the child attempts a more complex structure, such as a subordinate clause introduced by 'because', this may be the point at which syntax breaks down, articulation and fluency falter, and the child is unable to integrate the different aspects of language to produce a coherent message. Having said that, there may still be no outward signs of brain damage or intellectual defect in children so affected.

In chapter 2 we set out the syntactic patterns which children can be expected to control at the different stages and a summary is provided in table 3.5. Using this framework as a series of bench-marks, it should be possible to compare an individual child's level of grammatical awareness with the normal level of sentence patterning produced by children of the same age. Children delayed by more than one year, or who show confused patterns of sentence structure, should be referred on to the speech therapist for advice.

Vocabulary

It is in the area of vocabulary that some children's language difficulties are highlighted. Children may have clear articulation and use a range of sentence structures, but appear to be unable to store words or to recover them from memory when needed. We have said that simply counting the number of words children have in their vocabularies is less revealing than discovering the range of uses to which they are put. For example, it may be that a child has a

Table 3.5 *Summary of sentence structures at different stages of grammatical development*

Age of child (in months)	Stage	Typical sentence patterns
9 to 18	I (one element)	'car', 'doggy', 'cup', 'more', 'Mummy', 'there'
18 to 24	II (two elements)	'Daddy car', 'more biccy', 'where pussy', 'no drink', 'hat off', 'want Mummy'
24 to 30	III (three elements)	'Where my dolly', 'I eated my dinner', 'My teddy gone now', 'Give ball Dada'
30 to 36	IV (four elements)	'Can you get it', 'Grandma gone down the shop', 'We going swimming in a minute'
36 to 42	V (complex sentences)	'We went to the park and we had a ride on the swing and I fell off'

persistent difficulty in using verbs – the 'action' words of language. Since all sentences require a verb the child with few to utilise is likely, as a consequence, to have severe problems in developing syntax patterns. What of the child who produces sentences like this – 'That thing over there isn't doing what it should do because they're not supposed to do things like that'? This is a complex sentence which lacks semantic specificity, another kind of 'empty language'. The child is unable to particularise the meaning, to say distinctly and precisely what is meant, because of a narrow vocabulary range.

> *At nine years, Dean's specific language problem was that he could not find the exact word he wanted to express an idea. This difficulty in retrieving words out of memory store could be demonstrated very clearly by asking Dean to give the names of some everyday objects shown on picture cards. In many instances he would have to talk around an item, being unable to come up with the name itself. He had difficulty remembering the names of colours, days of the week, months of the year, animals, and the names of familiar people (see table 3.6). It could be that he had not met some of these particular words before, but word-finding difficulties are rarely a result of lack of experience. In all other respects – intelligence, physical senses, motor skills – a child with word-finding problems may be perfectly ordinary. Needless to say, such problems can seriously interfere with a child's ability to communicate, not least of all in terms of confidence.*

Table 3.6 *Examples of a child's word-finding difficulties in response to picture stimuli*

Picture stimulus	Child's response
television	thing you have; radio, aerial
lorry	bus
magician's wand	that's his hold thing
duck	water bird
nose	a breathing
axe	tree chopper
diver	undersea man
hanger	a clothes up tidy
waterfall	fish step
matches	got fire in them
church	go get married
watering can	water flower
clutch pedal	you hop on it
drill	hole maker
tomato	a round red

Specific reading and writing difficulties

Most of what we have to say in this book concerns the development of oral language. The *primary* functions of language we have described in terms of social interaction with others, communicating feelings, wishes, demands, and information. Through oral language children discover, manipulate and categorise their environment. Spoken language is the vehicle of discussion, reflection and analysis. As soon as the child arrives in school, these primary functions of spoken language are developed further, as well as being extended into a quite different mode. In school, the child is asked to apply verbal knowledge, skills and strategies to written language. Reading and writing are *secondary* language processes which require a different kind of language awareness from the child. In speech, the child acquires the rules which govern sounds, grammar and word meanings, almost without conscious awareness: there is often no need to think about the system we use. In learning written language the child has to think consciously about the rules for constructing and recognising a message in print. It is at this point, when a child encounters the printed language code, that difficulties may arise.

Specific reading and writing difficulties are sometimes described by the medical-sounding label 'dyslexia'. However, the presence of any physical factors such as hearing or visual loss, or any overt symptoms of brain damage, are usually discounted before children are described as 'dyslexic'. In fact, the characteristic picture is one of a bright child from a supportive family, with no explanation for an apparently surprising inability to read or spell. Children are sometimes said to be unable to read *because they are 'dyslexic'*. However, this is akin to saying a child is ill because he does not feel well. The term 'dyslexia' only means that, for some inexplicable reason, a child has reading difficulties. This is not to say that all children who suffer from dyslexia share the same problems or can be 'treated' in the same way.

Recently, writers such as Vellutino (1979) and Snowling (1985) have suggested that dyslexia is really an extension of a child's earlier difficulties in oral language processes. The child's spoken language problems may have gone unrecognised, but later make it difficult for dealing with other language forms, such as print. What kind of language-processing difficulties are thought to create later difficulties in reading and spelling? In the book edited by Snowling (1985) a range of verbal deficits are referred to, ranging from the gross to the particular. A child might have a general inability to organise information properly, so that the whole of the school experience is bewildering, including the first efforts to teach letters and words. We can predict that where children have a limited fund of vocabulary at their disposal, immature sentence patterns and a lack of experience in using language to think, categorise and explore relationships between events in the world, then they will be less prepared to tackle the linguistic puzzles presented by print.

However, dyslexia theorists tend to pin-point some very specific verbal processes as underlying reading difficulties. These usually involve dealing with the sound (or phonemic) units of speech. There is a lot of evidence to suggest that children who can perform sound segmentation tasks make good readers. Typical tasks include tapping out individual sounds in syllables (f-a-t), blending sounds together (br+ing = bring), adding or subtracting sounds (s+pin = spin, spin−s = pin), exchanging initial sounds in two words to make a spoonerism (car park, par cark), discriminating between like-sounding words (wig, big), detecting a word which does not rhyme (hat, cat, hit), and identifying alliteration (see, sock, sun). Quite often these tasks are presented in isolation from an actual reading task and there are a number of ways in which a child can find them difficult: perceiving the sound differences, pronouncing the sound contrasts, or simply remembering them. 'Dyslexic' children are thought to have problems in segmenting phonemes at a critical time when these skills are required for learning to read (Bryant and Bradley, 1985).

What is the significance of these sound skills for reading? Why should children who are good at categorising and recognising sounds, rhymes, and alliteration become better spellers and readers? A sound or phonic-based view of reading suggests that children need to know two things in order to begin to read. The first insight is that our spoken language can be split up into separate units such as phonemes, words, and sentences. The second insight is that these spoken features correspond roughly to units that can be written down and then read. So, the child must be aware that a word like 'cat' has three segments. Each segment can be represented by a letter and the child uses this knowledge to convert the written word into a series of spoken sounds – 'kuh-ah-tuh'. In this way a child can identify unfamiliar words by hearing how the word is pronounced. Most children naturally use a phonic strategy when they try to spell a new word. Some of the mistakes children make, such as writing 'apul' for 'apple', demonstrate the child's method of breaking a word up into sound segments in order to spell it. Of course, not all words can be encoded, or decoded, correctly using sound strategies. However, the argument is made that children can learn the common spelling patterns in words such as 'light', 'fight', and 'sight', by recognising similarities in the word sounds (Bryant and Bradley, 1985).

Not everyone agrees that reading failure can be explained simply in terms of lack of sensitivity to sounds in words. Researchers continue to look for the 'missing link' which accounts for reading difficulties. Some theorists pin their hopes on defects in visual perception, eye movements or high-level processes such as comprehension of word meanings. It is safe to assume that no one, single factor will have the power to account for all the problems children may experience in learning to read. Reading is a highly complex intellectual activity requiring a multiplicity of skills. In the language model put forward in chapter 2 (figure 2.1), sounds occupy a peripheral position. It could be argued, just as plausibly, that other aspects of language are equally important to reading as sounds. A child's knowledge of sentence structure helps to predict the kind of words to be found at a particular point in the sentence frame. So too, the child may be helped to predict meaning by using picture clues, story line, sensible guess work and cross checking. All of these information sources help a child to read. Some of the clues lie in the letters and sounds on the page. Other clues lie in the reader's own knowledge and experience. Children with limited spoken language may be at a disadvantage on both counts as they approach the reading task.

Although we cannot predict accurately in every case, it is fair to assume that many children with early difficulties in acquiring the *primary* spoken language will have later problems in learning to read and write. It is important, then, that details of any child known to the speech therapist are passed on to teaching staff and reading progress is monitored carefully. Conversely, there should be no complacency about children who appear to be slow in developing literacy. By the age of seven, at the latest, children who have fallen behind in their reading progress should be referred to a reading specialist, support teacher, or educational psychologist for advice and help. Children who experience more severe language delay or disorder will undoubtedly face problems in reading and writing. An underlying inability to use spoken language will hinder progress in all areas of verbal skill, such as reading, and this has important implications for linking approaches to language and literacy in school.

PROFESSIONAL ROLES

This chapter has tried to cover the wide variety of ways in which the processes of normal language development may be disrupted. Using the framework of normal speech and language acquisition described in chapter 2, we have set out the likely effects of factors such as hearing loss, visual or motor impairment, learning, and social and emotional difficulties, upon the child's development of speech and language. We have tried to avoid using categories and labels, in order to move the focus of interest away from the child's handicap towards the child and the learning environment. It should always be borne in mind that children's difficulties rarely occur in just one dimension. Problems tend to go together and spill over into other areas of development. There will be few children with severe hearing losses, to take an example, who do not also experience social and emotional setbacks and whose interactions with others are not interfered with.

We hope that teachers will be prompted to discover something of every child's individual capabilities and limitations. The children at greatest risk in ordinary classrooms are not necessarily those with the most severe and obvious handicaps, because these may have been discovered early and the children given a lot of help. Perhaps we ought to pay greatest attention to the child with a small degree of hearing loss, together with a slight visual impairment, minor motor problems, occasional asthma, and with a history of epileptic fits. This is the more typical, albeit more frequently overlooked, child with special needs. In speech and language terms, enormity of handicap in one dimension is probably less significant than minor difficulties in a number of dimensions.

In this final section we shall be summarising the professional responsibilities of different agencies involved with children who have communication difficulties, and with whom teachers may have contact. We shall also be defining the teacher's own responsibilities in the identification and assessment process.

The Health Visitor

At the pre-school stage the responsibility for early identification of children with special needs in speech and language lies mainly with community health services. Health Visitors see families with young children periodically to give advice on care and management, and to make developmental observations. They are often the first professionals to whom parents express their concerns, they have oversight of siblings and are able to link up with other medical agencies. Their continuity of contact with the family puts them in a good position to recognise when a child is slow to develop speech, for example. Health Visitors screen all babies at around eight months for hearing, vision and general development. The kind of checklist sometimes used by Health Visitors as a basis for observing young children is included in Appendix 1, and this gives some idea of the factors which can be looked for early on to identify potential problems in speech and language.

The Medical Officer

There are basically two kinds of medical provision for children – treatment services provided by hospitals and the primary care team (which includes the GP), and preventative services within the community. It could be said that all doctors are concerned with detecting developmental problems from the time of birth onwards. However, the precise role of doctors varies widely from one health district to another. Doctors who are likely to be involved in identifying children with special needs in speech and language are the Clinical Medical Officers who work in well-baby clinics, schools, and other community services. Medical Officers play a key role in identifying early difficulties both in pre-school child health clinics and on school entry, when most children are medically examined. Children who are identified as having abnormalities or possible developmental delay may be referred on to Senior Clinical Medical Officers or consultant paediatricians for further investigation. Senior Clinical Medical Officers liaise between hospital services and the education authority. They will indicate the significance of any medical findings for later educational provision. In some areas, Health Visitors who are concerned at a child's late development of speech refer directly to a Senior Clinical Medical Officer for a more detailed examination. Medical Officers who work in the community contribute not only to early screening, but also to the multi-professional assessment of children whose needs may require special educational help, and to the continual monitoring and review of children once they are in school.

The Speech Therapist

Speech Therapists are responsible for the assessment, diagnosis and treatment of communication problems, in the widest sense of the term. They usually work for a Health Authority, but accept referrals from parents, teachers and other professionals, as well as doctors. Speech Therapists are able to give a detailed assessment of a child's speech and language abilities; they may organise further investigations, such as a hearing test, or an X-ray of the palate; and carry out a programme of treatment. Speech Therapists are increasingly aware of the need to work in close collaboration with parents and other professionals. They have a role to play in passing on information and skills to other people concerned with the child.

The view of Speech Therapists 'correcting' a child's speech articulation problem on weekly visits to an outpatient's clinic is an outdated one. Speech Therapists make much more important contributions to the overall management of communication difficulties. They will make valuable suggestions for both parents and teachers to use in the natural learning contexts of the home and school. Increasingly, Speech Therapists are working in partnership with teachers and parents, helping to devise strategies which enable the child to take part in the communication environment.

The Educational Psychologist

Educational Psychologists have a training in child psychology as well as in teaching and usually lay claim to a wide experience of normal children as well as those with developmental and learning difficulties. Employed by the local education authority, Educational Psychologists usually visit a group of ordinary and special schools as well as providing a service to the children and families who live in an area. Most Educational Psychologists are competent family counsellors and would be able to devise ways of helping parents deal with a behaviour problem, for example, at home. At the classroom level, most Educational Psychologists share the teacher's point of view and may be able to suggest ways of working with an individual or group. Most important of all, Educational Psychologists are officers of the local authority, sharing some of the responsibility for decision making and policy. As such they are able to advise on the availability of resources to schools, and take a key role in identifying and planning for children with special needs. In line with the 1981 Education Act, many Educational Psychologists co-ordinate the processes through which a child's special needs may be highlighted and appropriate educational provision made. All teachers should have access to the Educational Psychologist who visits the school in order to discuss any concerns about individual children, their families, or the learning environment.

The teacher

The ordinary class teacher has a major contribution to make to the processes of identifying children with special communication needs and devising an appropriate teaching curriculum. When children are helped within a mainstream class it falls largely to the class teacher to ask other support agencies for advice at the appropriate time, and to plan, monitor, and evaluate the child's learning experience. Not least of all, it is the teacher's responsibility to keep parents in touch with developments in school and to involve them in the learning process. The Warnock Report, and the 1981 Education Act which followed it, have both been influential in shaping current attitudes and working practice. We shall highlight some of the major implications of this legislation in relation to children with communication difficulties and the class teachers who have day-to-day responsibility for them.

The 1981 Education Act[1] has placed a general duty on schools to be more aware of children with special needs. A special educational need is to be defined, not in terms of the child's category of handicap, but in terms of whatever learning obstacles the child has to overcome. Teachers should have found this chapter useful in outlining how a learning obstacle, such as hearing loss or visual impairment, arises, what implications such obstacles hold for development, and how they may be identified. We have said that approximately ten per cent of all children have a language handicap which is serious enough to warrant special help. So it is incumbent upon schools to have efficient screening and monitoring processes of their own, which can identify children hitherto unrecognised. In Appendix 1 we have provided just such a screening profile which outlines the kinds of factors teachers should be alert to in children who may give rise for concern. Many teachers find these profiles of

---

[1]The legislation discussed in this chapter applies in England, Wales and Northern Ireland. Different legislation applies in Scotland as a result of the Education (Scotland) Act 1981 and its governing regulations (1982). For details of the Scottish Act see (MacKay (1986) or Ward (1985).

communication skills helpful in guiding their own informal observations of children. Profiles can help the teacher plan a teaching programme geared to the child's specific strengths and weaknesses. They are also helpful as a basis for continual record keeping over a long period of time.

Informal and formal procedures

The most complex proposals in the 1981 Education Act concern the *formal* procedures whereby a full, multi-professional assessment of a child's needs is made, leading to a 'statement'. However, Circular 1/83, which accompanies the Act, gives a lot of advice to schools about the *informal* stages of assessment and consultation. Schools are asked to keep clear and effective lines of communication with outside agencies. When a child comes into school with a *known* language difficulty, contact with supporting professionals, such as the speech therapist, should be established. If a teacher *becomes* concerned about a child with a speech problem, both parent and head teacher should be told, as soon as possible. Circular 1/83 suggests that schools should be frank and open with parents, sharing any misgivings before a situation becomes critical. Similarly, schools should know whom to call on for advice and help. Every school has access to a school nurse, school doctor, and Educational psychologist. Circular 1/83 describes what it calls a 'progressive extension of professional involvement', starting with the class teacher, then the head, and on to health and psychological services, perhaps eventually involving more specialist agencies, such as a hospital consultant. A note should be made in the child's records at the time any difficulties were identified, of whom the school referred on to, and what was done to help.

Formal procedures under the 1981 Education Act are usually started when there are grounds for believing that a child has special needs which cannot be met within the resources normally available to the ordinary school. Obviously, this will vary from area to area, depending on the kind of resources schools can call upon. In some authorities all schools have access to remedial or language support teachers, and to speech therapists. If a child's needs cannot be met from the support readily available to the school, the formal statutory procedures are initiated to ascertain as fully as possible what the child's needs are and how they might be met. The child who requires classroom help additional to that already available, or the child who would benefit from more specialist teaching in a unit for children with communication difficulties, or the child who requires a special school environment, should all be formally assessed and a 'statement' issued.

The Local Education Authority collects the views of parents, teacher, medical officer, psychologist and any other professional involved with the child, such as a speech therapist. The formal procedures are technically complex and give parents the right to request or object to assessment, to seek independent advice, to be present at any examinations, and to receive copies of all professional advice submitted during the assessment process. There are statutory periods of notice at various points, and parents have rights of appeal. A statement, setting out the nature of the child's special needs and how the authority proposes to meet them, is usually only issued when all the participants, including the parents, are in agreement. Any extra or alternative provision, such as a special school, will be named in the statement, together with a date for review. The statement is meant to *protect* the present and future interests of the child whose needs are highlighted in the assessment partnership.

—4—
Language tests and language schemes

In this chapter we shall be passing a critical eye over some of the language assessment procedures which have been devised, toge- ther with a sample of the remedial packages which are available commercially. Up to this point we have discussed language acquisition within a framework of the normal developmental process. Similarly, the approach we have taken to children with language difficulties uses the parameters for describing communi- cation skills which have emerged from the study of normal development. No apology is made for this. The present state of the art is such that the most complete models which have been constructed to help us understand the sequence of language development, have centred upon *typical* children. These provide the best guidelines we have, at the moment, for describing the skills which are appropriate at a given age, the relative order in which skills are achieved, and what appear to be the natural learning steps to aim for in the teaching context. The teacher who has a clear understanding of the normal unfolding of language behaviour will be in a good position to organise a learning programme to meet a child's needs.

This is not to say that formal tests of language have no place. Used sensibly, and with an awareness of the particular possibilities or limitations inherent in test materials, they can be a source of helpful *supportive* information. There is a very wide range of assessment procedures available. Some tests help the teacher to describe more clearly a child's level of competence in a discrete area of language skill, such as comprehension of spoken vocabulary. Other tests provide descriptions of wider areas of development, for example, in summarising a child's expressive verbal abilities. Several batteries of language tests have been designed which tap contrasting areas of language skill within the same child, so that a profile of strengths and weaknesses is derived. Two broad approaches, norm-refer- enced and criterion-referenced, are used for assessing performance. In norm-referenced testing, the information yielded is in the form of a comparison: how well the test child has performed in relation to the average performance of children of the same chronological age. In criterion-referenced testing, the aim is to determine whether a child has attained a target behaviour within a sequence of skilled behaviours.

The selection of appropriate test materials will depend on the nature of the information required and the purposes for which it will be used. At a *macro* level, a psychologist might prefer to use a test which gives a general description of a child, for example, receptive language age. That measure might be more useful at an administrative stage, in arguing a case for further resources within a particular school. On the other hand, a teacher planning an educational programme would require observations at a *micro* level, using a form of assessment which reveals the fine grain of a child's language skill. In some contexts, both levels of assessment are useful, such as when a child's progress is evaluated over time and a general summary is required, leading to future teaching plans, when more specific objectives are set.

As a general consideration it should be noted that test materials, in themselves, cannot be expected to provide insights into a child's behaviour. They may help a teacher to confirm or reject a particular hypothesis. But if a teacher does not know what to look out for, or which questions to ask, then tests will not reveal useful data or workable solutions. Test procedures sample only a small part of a child's current functioning. There are great temptations to believe that tests somehow describe the whole child (IQ is a good example), and can predict how well a child will progress: neither, in fact, is the case. It is also tempting to consider assessment as a separate process from the business of teaching. However, when we come to consider commercially produced intervention kits, it is apparent that the most successful 'ready made' methods link observation and teaching closely together, so that the assessment process both informs, and arises out of, the teaching context.

NORM-REFERENCED TESTS

Most 'standardised' tests have at their core an assumption that abilities are evenly distributed across a population, such that an equal number of cases will fall above and below a statistical mean. Tests are constructed so that children's scores will spread out across this range. In using a standardised measure we expect half the children to whom it is applied to be below average. A 'below average' score on a measure of verbal skill should not be considered in the same light as, for example, 'below normal blood pressure'. It is a question of debate just how far below the average mark a child's scores have to fall before concern is registered. This will also vary according to the test materials. In all formal testing a small sample of a child's behaviour is taken, usually following a uniform procedure, and this is taken to be representative of an underlying trait. So, for example, by asking for responses to a selection of vocabulary pictures, the child's scores might be translated into a vocabulary age. The end product of this kind of language assessment, couched in terms like 'receptive quotient', gives few details which can be translated into teaching targets. On the other hand, aspects such as the child's concentration during the time of testing may have important implications for both the interpretation of results and future teaching plans.

There are several key questions which teachers need to ask themselves in relation to normative tests. The first question considers the *validity* of the materials. Validity is the degree to which a test measures what it sets out to measure. On an intuitive basis, teachers will be aware that a test which purports to measure vocabulary, and which demands written responses from the child, may well be testing spelling ability. Test compilers usually provide evidence that the test measures what it claims to measure, by carrying out a statistical analysis to see how the results achieved using one test correlate with the results achieved using another, similar test. Even when this sort of statistical analysis has been done, there is no guarantee that a test will reveal the same kind of information in different children. There is, in fact, a body of evidence which suggests that children with special needs, such as those with a hearing impairment, may use atypical strategies to solve test-puzzles, which casts doubt on the validity of measures such as reading age. In one instance, deaf children completed a reading test without reading (Webster, Wood, and Griffiths, 1981; Wood, Griffiths, and Webster, 1981). Teachers must always ask themselves, when thinking about using a test: 'What does this material really tell me?'

Subsequent questions that teachers might ask about tests include:
'What kind of theory lies behind the material?'
'What kind of practical information does the test reveal?'
'How was the test put together and what was the author's purpose?'
'Are the results easy to interpret?'
'Can the test be used a second time and will it give similar results?'
'Does the test procedure fit in with the teacher's way of working?'
'At what level of intervention is the test an effective tool?'

CRITERION-REFERENCED TESTS

In criterion-referenced tests the focus of interest is the individual's ability to reach specific goals: what a child can actually do in an area of skill such as language. Emphasis shifts away from individual differences and their relationship with the mean. It is the identification of learning or developmental criteria which is of interest, and the individual's performance relative to these. The use of standardised procedures with young children or children with special needs is often difficult. However, criterion-referenced approaches often do not require strict adherence to a uniform test procedure. Since the concern is whether a child has achieved specific skills, observations can be built up over time, in different contexts and can include the insights of important adults, particularly parents. Criterion-referenced tests can be thought of as providing a framework for systematic observation, within which the child's strengths and weaknesses can be discovered. Using such a framework, assessment can be continual and closely tied to the teaching context. Such tests usually provide a detailed profile of the skills or knowledge which have been mastered, or the level of competence reached in different skill areas. Armed with this kind of specific information about a child, the teacher is in a strong position to detail the future teaching targets at which to aim.

Where do criteria come from? In some cases the author of a test begins by scanning the developmental literature. There will be found the collective research evidence on the emergence of skills in a particular domain of behaviour during childhood. Some domains are better charted than others. A lot of evidence has been gathered together by linguists on the sequence of language acquisition in early childhood. On the other hand, language development beyond the age of about seven years is more complex and less well-documented. The learning steps through which children move are not so clearly defined. In the domain of reading, for example, there is less certainty about the significant skills which children need, the order in which these skills are acquired, and, consequently, priorities for teachers to consider.

With criterion-referenced tests teachers should ask themselves:
'Are the learning criteria derived from research evidence?'
'Do the skills which are profiled adequately cover the behaviour domain of interest?'
'Are the learning steps clearly defined and do they follow an ordered sequence?'
'Can the test information be easily translated into practical teaching targets?'

REVIEW OF TEST MATERIALS

This is not intended to be an exhaustive review. The aim is to examine a representative selection of materials, to discuss purpose, form and utility of procedures, and to relate the whole to the areas of language study described in figure 2.1.

Symbolic Play Test (Lowe and Costello, 1976)

This is a test developed for children aged from one to three years which can be used by teachers to assess early symbolic understanding and concept formation. It is based on observations of representational play in young children and gives an age level for symbolic understanding in relation to small toys. Miniature toys, such as a bed, pillow, blanket, and doll, are presented in a given sequence, without verbal instructions. The child's response to the play material, in relating the doll to the bed, for example, indicates the level of symbolic awareness. It would be helpful to support the test responses with observations from wider play contexts, such as the home or a toddler group. The test provides structured criteria for observing early play: important, when children have language delays, in determining whether the child can represent the world in toy (pre-word) symbols. In chapter 5 we consider the selection of appropriate play resources and the significance of play in the fostering of receptive and expressive language. An informal, Piagetian-based, framework is discussed.

Edinburgh Articulation Test (Anthony et al., 1971)

A number of tests have been designed to give a picture of the developing phonology of young children, an aspect of language which occupies the left-hand side of figure 2.1. Such tests are of more immediate value to the speech therapist and require specialist knowledge in phonetic transcription and interpretation. The Edinburgh test analyses the articulation of consonant sounds rather than vowels (which are felt to give less reliable indications of overall speech mastery), in the speech of three- to six-year-olds. It is based on existing research knowledge of normal phonological development. Articulation is said to approximate adult speech in most respects by the age of six. A set of coloured pictures is presented to the child as part of a naming game, one word per illustration. Examples such as monkey, fish, umbrella, chimney, garage, bottle, finger, and scissors were selected because of their familiarity, the phonological information revealed, and the power they gave to discriminate between normal and speech-delayed children. The child's responses are used for both qualitative and quantitative analysis of the sound system. Attempts at a word with fricative sounds, such as the 'f' in feather, can be used to identify speech patterns associated, for example, with a high frequency hearing loss. The quantitative score is calculated by adding correct items and then comparing an individual's total score with the standardisation data derived from a sample of 510 children. An 'articulation age' of one year behind chronological age is said to be the point to register concern. For the specialist, useful descriptive information is given, when a therapy programme is planned. What is not considered in this test, is *how* adults can interact with children in order to help speech intelligibility: the strategies for communicative interaction.

Test for auditory comprehension of language (Carrow, 1973)

There is a wide range of assessment procedures designed to assess what has been described as the central organising principles of grammar, but these vary greatly in range and depth. The Carrow test is for use by teachers and language specialists with children from three to seven years of age. The material consists of 101 items, each requiring a choice, by pointing, between three black and white pictures. The stimulus varies from individual verbs, such as 'eating', to full sentences such as 'The boy is at the side of the car', with the target picture illustrating the linguistic form being tested. A child can be given a developmental level of comprehension in comparison with test norms. Information on the test sheet gives age levels at which 75 per cent and 90 per cent of children pass each item. There are also diagnostic guidelines for identifying points of grammar which are causing comprehension problems, so that a programme can be closely tailored to the child's needs. The structures in the test are not ordered in terms of level of difficulty, but are grouped according to structural type, such as pronouns, verb tenses, prepositions, adjectives, adverbs, word suffixes, and syntax forms.

Although the Carrow test gives a useful profile of language comprehension, there are several criticisms of the material. The static line drawings do not always represent the language stimuli, such as action verbs, very clearly. The lack of a developmental sequence in the test items leaves some uncertainty about the relative importance of any gaps in a child's profile, and what to aim for in a teaching programme. In common with most descriptive measures, no strategies for teaching are given.

Test for Reception of Grammar (Bishop, 1983)

TROG is an individually administered test, suitable for the age range 4–13 years, which can be used by teachers to discover the range of grammatical contrasts understood by the child. There are three parallel forms of the test, each containing 40 items, divided into ten blocks. Each block tests comprehension of one type of grammatical contrast, such as negative/affirmative, singular/plural, active/passive, pronouns in subject/object position, and comparatives. Items are preceded by a vocabulary check to ensure that the child understands the nouns, verbs, and adjectives to be used. The child is given an array of four pictures whilst a sentence, such as 'The knife is longer than the pencil', or 'The dog is not drinking', is spoken. The child indicates, by pointing, which picture corresponds to the test sentence. TROG has been standardised so that age equivalents can be calculated for each child's total score. Specific areas of comprehension failure are also highlighted. This is a useful evaluative procedure, so long as the examiner can relate the findings to a developmental perspective.

Language Assessment, Remediation, and Screening Procedure
(Crystal, Fletcher, and Garman, 1976)

LARSP is a criterion-referenced profile for analysing the grammar of spoken language. This complex and time-consuming procedure requires training to administer. Derived from the literature of normal child language development, LARSP provides a framework for making a comprehensive description of a child's (or adult's) syntactic output, which is plotted on a profile chart. To begin with, a 15- to 30-minute sample of free conversation is recorded and transcribed. The early sections of the profile chart account for interactive processes between child and adult, as well as unanalysed sentences, but the central and most useful section concerns the analysis of sentence structure. LARSP hypothesises a set of seven syntactic stages through which children progress towards the adult language. (See discussion of grammatical development in chapter 2 for details of stages.) LARSP classifies the structures which operate at each stage and gives an approximate age when new patterns of language are likely to occur. Central to this approach is the idea that every sentence has a distribution of complexity which can be broken down according to the various levels within the syntactic profile. In broad terms three kinds of sentence structure are recognised: patterns of clause structure, word structure, and sentence connection. Analysis of a subject's sentences proceeds through a series of checks or 'scans'. Scan 3, for example, notes any connecting devices between sentences, such as 'however', or 'actually'. Features which interrelate clauses or extend sentence sequences, such as the conjunction 'and', are identified in scan 4. The analysis of individual clause patterns begins at scan 5, when features such as subject, verb, adverb are identified. Scan 6 establishes phrase structures whilst scan 7 records the various types of modifications as words are put together.

In the LARSP analysis each instance of a particular grammatical feature can be tabulated within a developmental framework. Assuming that an adequate sample can be obtained in the first place, the weakness of this approach is that everything has to be counted, however insignificant, and a reduction to the most salient features would be desirable. For those who master it, LARSP helps to identify areas of a child's grammar which are well established, still emerging, or requiring specific remediation. As such it is probably most useful to specialists working with children who have severe language delays or disorders, where strengths and weaknesses need to be carefully pin-pointed, and when a systematic programme of remediation is planned. The clear definition LARSP gives both to patterns of grammar as they unfold, and across the range of expressive syntax, is perhaps its greatest asset.

British Picture Vocabulary Scales (Dunn, Dunn, and Whetton, 1981)

As we have mentioned previously the number of words in a child's vocabulary was at one time held to be a good measure of a child's development in general, and semantic development in particular (the aspect of language concerned with meaning, which occupies the right-hand side of the diagram in figure 2.1.) It is now recognised that the range and flexibility of the vocabulary a child employs is more important than a static word count; and, furthermore, word meanings cannot be isolated from the social context in which words are used. For these reasons, vocabulary tests are suspect as screening measures. The BPVS is a typical test of receptive vocabulary, standardised for the age range two and a half to eighteen years. It is presented in short or long form, each version giving a graded series of choices from four black and white pictures, with a single stimulus word requiring a pointing response. The test is simple to administer and score, but the information derived is limited. Correct responses to items such as 'bucket', 'ankle', 'bee', 'socket', 'dangerous', 'money' are totalled to give a receptive vocabulary age. How the latter figure relates to the child's functional understanding and use of vocabulary, or to the child's wider abilities, is unclear.

Reynell Developmental Language Scales – revised edition (Reynell, 1977)

The Reynell test is probably the most widely used language assessment measure amongst speech therapists in the United Kingdom. The test is standardised for one- to seven-year-olds, but is most useful for children between the ages of two and four years with separate directions for hearing-impaired and physically-handicapped subjects. This is one of several test batteries which aim to give a comprehensive picture of the child's linguistic functioning, including aspects of cognitive skill important for language development. The theoretical background to the scales has been described in some detail by Reynell (1969), and there are a number of parallels with the Soviet accounts of development discussed in chapter 2. For example, Reynell relates the early stages of attention, object recognition, and symbolic play to corresponding growth in the child's verbal understanding and expressive ability. She suggests, as did Luria (1961) and Vygotsky (1962), that at the age of about five years, language becomes internalised in order to facilitate thinking and regulate the child's behaviour. The Reynell test consists of a 'verbal comprehension' and an 'expressive language' scale. The former consists of a selection of life-size objects and miniature toys, which are presented to the child with increasingly complex spoken instructions. In the early stages the child might be asked 'Where is the ball?'; an intermediate task might include 'Put the spoon in the cup'; whilst a later example is 'Put all the white pigs round the outside of the field.' The expressive scale has three sections. The first notes vocalisations, babble, and recognisable words. The second assesses word knowledge through objects, pictures, and questions. The third appraises creative use of language in describing pictures.

The Reynell scales give contrasting summaries of a child's receptive and expressive language maturity, which can be an important diagnostic indicator pointing to where a child's major problems lie. The scales have been criticised by linguists, such as Crystal, Fletcher, and Garman (1976), on the grounds of selectivity. The expressive scale is concerned more with the developments in length and quantity of a child's utterances, rather than growing sophistication in structural features. How much the test itself reveals in terms of teaching targets is questionable, and it is perhaps most valuable as a screening device, or in monitoring children's progress over time. In fact, a teaching programme for children with language disabilities has evolved from the Reynell scales, aimed at establishing attention control, the transfer of focus, and early concept formation. Some aspects of this work are discussed in chapter 5, when attention and listening skills are examined further, and later in this chapter.

Illinois Test of Psycholinguistic Abilities – revised edition (Kirk, McCarthy and Kirk, 1968)

The ITPA is an example of a procedure which aims to assess a broad spectrum of cognitive abilities, including auditory and visual perception, memory, sequencing, and symbolic understanding. It is argued that by identifying and treating weak cognitive processes, language skills can be improved. The ITPA is a standardised battery for children from two to ten years, which is demanding to administer. Originally, the starting point for the test was a model of all the processes involved in understanding and speaking a language, proposed by communication engineers. The model distinguishes three dimensions. The first concerns *channels of communication*: the sensory routes through which language flows. For example, the auditory–vocal channel takes input through the ear and gives a verbal response. A second dimension concerns *levels of organisation*. The reference is to the habits of communication. The 'representational level' requires the inner manipulation of meaningful symbols, whilst the 'automatic level' is concerned with highly organised chains of responses. The third dimension is to do with *psycholinguistic processes*. The distinction here is between processes of understanding and expression and the organising processes which mediate between input and output. The ITPA material itself consists of ten subtests, which are shown in table 4.1. Each of the subtests yields a raw score, language age or standard score, together with a total 'psycholinguistic age' for the whole.

The ITPA is valued by language specialists because it gives a breakdown of the cognitive processes important for language: several remedial programmes have been designed around the ITPA profile. (See discussion of GOAL later in this chapter.) The question has sometimes been raised whether the cognitive abilities assessed in the ITPA procedure may be the cause of language disorders, or whether they result from language difficulties in the first place. The results of studies which have evaluated 'psycholinguistic training' are equivocal. Some researchers feel the battery omits specifically linguistic aspects, such as syntax; whilst others feel its strength lies in the broader approach taken to language within a cognitive framework. In the light of more recent work in child language development the theoretical model on which ITPA was based is outdated.

Aston Index (Newton and Thomson, 1976)

Although the Aston Index promotes itself as a classroom test for screening and diagnosing language difficulties, in fact the material is focussed on reading and writing. It is for use by teachers and speech therapists with subjects aged 5 to 14 years, and is said to identify children with a wide range of special needs, including language disorders and dyslexia. The test is not underpinned by any particular theory or model and is really a battery of miscellan-

Table 4.1 *Subtests of the Illinois Test of Psycholinguistic Abilities – Revised Edition* (Kirk, McCarthy, and Kirk, 1968)

Subject	Test description
Auditory reception	Simple questions (do dogs eat?)
Visual reception	Matching pictures which belong to the same category (shoes)
Auditory association	Verbal analogies (soup is hot, icecream is ...)
Visual association	Relating pictures (hammer with nail)
Verbal expression	Expressing ideas in speech (child has to talk about pictures showing ball, brick, etc.)
Manual expression	Miming appropriate actions to pictures (telephone, guitar)
Grammatical closure	Finishing incomplete statements to test grammar (This dog likes to bark; here he is ...)
Visual closure	Identifying common objects which are incomplete and partially hidden amongst others
Auditory memory	Recalling a series of numbers in the order given
Visual memory	Reproducing a series of abstract symbols

eous items which are more or less related to language, many of them taken from standardised intelligence scales. Level 1, for children between five and seven years, includes the Goodenough Draw-a-Man Test, copying name, copying geometric designs, left/right discrimination, tests of sound discrimination, blending, and sequencing, and tests of vocabulary and picture recognition. This level of the test, concerned as it is with a range of skills often heralded to be *prerequisite* to literacy, can be used as a screening measure. Level 2, for children over the age of seven years, comprises several of the earlier vocabulary, laterality, drawing, copying, and auditory tests; together with the Schonell reading and spelling tests; a free writing test; and a measure of grapheme/phoneme awareness. From this information an ability profile is built up for each child, and there are data for comparison of each subtest score with the standardisation sample.

In chapter 3 we pointed out that specific reading and writing difficulties (sometimes described by the term 'dyslexia') encompass a broad spectrum of language processing difficulties, from the gross to the particular. Some dyslexia theorists ascribe literacy problems to earlier spoken language immaturity, for example, a limited range of vocabulary. Others pin-point specific sound segmentation deficits, such as phonic blending. The Aston Index reflects the character of much dyslexia research, since we are talking about a composite group of learning difficulties in a diverse population of children whose common feature is the fact of poor school achievement. It is not surprising, therefore, that evidence is lacking on the ability of the Aston Index to *predict* those children who may have learning difficulties later on, given that there is little agreement over what constitutes the prerequisite skills for literacy. However, the battery does provide an easily administered screening test of current functioning in a wide range of skill areas important in the classroom.

Linguistic Awareness in Reading Readiness Test (Downing, Ayers and Schaefer, 1983)

LARR is a series of group tests for children in the first two years of infant schooling. Almost all of the existing tests of 'reading readiness' are concerned with the subskills of reading, such as visual perception and letter-name knowledge. (See, for example, the Aston Index.) In contrast, LARR focuses on the linguistic concepts and awareness of language which the child brings to reading tasks. Standardisation of the scale is still in the experimental stage, and the test is probably best used descriptively to evaluate children's awareness of the range of functions and features of written language. Part 1 of the LARR scale, 'Recognising literacy behaviour', examines the child's understanding of the nature of literacy – does the child know the difference between reading and writing, and whether it is the text or the pictures which are 'read'? Part 2, 'Understanding literacy functions', deals with the communicative intentions of different forms of text – does the child know that people read in order to find out when the the bus goes, how to build a model or bake a cake, and to enjoy a story? Part 3, 'Technical language of literacy', tests knowledge of terms such as 'letter', 'top line', 'word' or 'sentence'. Essentially, LARR assesses the child's inferences about print. Good predictive validity is claimed (the extent to which it predicts children's later achievements in reading). However, since a sophisticated level of language is assumed in following the instructions which accompany the test, children with mature linguistic understanding may do better on the test for that reason, rather than because LARR is a valid measure of conceptual readiness for reading.

THE ROLE OF LANGUAGE SCHEMES

The teacher who has some responsibility for meeting the needs of a group of children with communication difficulties may wish to examine the range of commercially produced kits or schemes: a growth area for publishers. Some of these materials are based on a particular theory of language development and may follow an assessment procedure constructed around the same model. Other materials have no theoretical underpinning and simply provide resources for language activities which have emerged from classroom practice. The emphasis of almost all language schemes is upon fostering expressive language. Usually, published materials are more suitable for individual and small group work, rather than general class use. The accommodation of special materials within the mainstream curriculum requires careful classroom management, and is discussed in chapter 5.

Before teachers commit themselves to a particular formal programme, a number of questions should be asked:
'What is the author's rationale for the scheme?'
'How far does the scheme echo what we know of the process of language development?'
'Will the material arouse interest in the children who are going to use it?'
'Does the style of teaching fit the teacher's own philosophy?'
'Can the scheme be incorporated, in time allocation, for example, with the day-to-day activities of a class?'

In our view, teachers should be careful not to become dependent on schemes in their approach to language. Published kits may be a useful source of suggestions which the teacher can develop. On the other hand, informal and spontaneous opportunities for exploring language often appear to be the most fruitful. In this book we have placed a lot of emphasis on the strategies that adults adopt, within a shared social context of language interaction, which provide the linguistic evidence from which children learn. In this natural learning paradigm the child is an active discoverer, initiating exchanges with adults who facilitate the child's thinking by a process of negotiation. The child's purposeful, hypothesis-testing approach to the world needs to be sustained. When adults try to teach language directly, moving the focus of communication away from the sharing of meaning towards the form of language, then language learning may falter.

A review of twenty-four language intervention programmes which focus on the early production and comprehension of spoken language has been given by Harris (1984). He shares the view expressed here, that language cannot be dispensed bit-by-bit from a teaching package devoid of a social context and in which the child is put in the position of passive respondent to the adults' demands. Ultimately, it is the quality of the child's linguistic interactions which appears to be the most important factor. The role which formal materials could play in this process is a supportive one, providing ready-made social contexts, within which social interaction can take place.

What kind of relationship should there be between testing and teaching? For the teacher, assessment is intimately linked with the setting of appropriate targets for the child, within a sequence of learning steps. For that reason, criterion-referenced tests are more helpful in helping to plan appropriate learning experiences, whilst norm-referenced tests are useful in measuring the outcome of any remedial teaching. There are a few published materials which bridge the gap between appraisal and language intervention, providing assessment profiles within which a child can be located, leading on to flexible strategies which can be implemented as part of the teaching process, together with continuing opportunities for evaluation of teaching outcomes.

REVIEW OF LANGUAGE KITS

A small selection of the vast array of published materials is reviewed here, the intention being to make a brief representative survey. Attention is paid to rationale, quality and utility, rather than to aspects such as value for money. For further details about materials designed for teaching sequencing, visuo-motor skills, and specific concepts, such as size or quantity, see Cooke and Williams (1985). *Ways and Means*, published by Somerset Education Authority (1978), also provides a useful review of materials for use with language delayed children.

The First Words Language Programme and Two Words Together
(Gillham, 1979, 1983)

These two books present programmes developed for use by parents or teachers with young children who have severe language delays, with the specific objectives of establishing single and double-element utterances. The first programme begins at the point where the child is attempting a few words, or has a small vocabulary range with significant gaps. A list of 100 words derived from a study of the early vocabulary of a sample of 14 babies is provided. As in the Nelson (1973) study referred to in chapter 2, the first words most frequently used by infants refer to people and objects around them, such as 'Mummy', 'shoe', and 'bath'. This list is used as the basis for a picture and object library. Having recorded a child's existing vocabulary, target words are selected according to the child's interests and developmental level. A variety of direct and informal teaching methods is described, including a viewer box which lights up pictures of objects, and puppets which demonstrate an action. The second programme uses card materials and cartoon character topic books to illustrate two-word sentences, such as 'dry toes', 'balloon bang', and 'wipe bottom', derived from records kept by 15 mothers of their children's first 50 word combinations. The value of both programmes lies in the clearly delineated teaching steps, target word lists, suggestions for setting objectives, and recording and evaluating progress. The books are particularly helpful in the very early stages and demonstrate that systematic teaching can also include natural and spontaneous learning contexts.

Helping Language Development (Cooper et al., 1978)

The authors describe this as a developmental language programme which is designed for children from two years upwards with language handicaps, based on the stages of symbolic understanding described by Reynell. Following activities directed at basic attention control, discussed in chapter 5, visual perception and motor skills are fostered using materials such as jigsaws and matched shapes. Work on concept formation proceeds through colours, sorting objects according to colour, size and type, categorisation by use, such as 'things for eating', concepts of size and quantity, and finally, positional concepts such as 'behind', 'under', and 'in-front'. Symbolic understanding is fostered through play, beginning with normal size objects, such as cups and spoons. Large doll play leads to activities with smaller toys, followed by the matching of toys to pictures, and eventually, gestures and words to pictures. Spoken language is taught in a similar sequential way, starting with the comprehension of one object related to another: 'Put the spoon in the box.' Teachers are encouraged to develop expressive language by expanding children's utterances, providing model sentences for completion, and direct questioning. Evaluation of the programme suggests that an integrated approach, where activities are directed towards cognitive as well as linguistic skills, may be very effective with young children.

Jim's People (Thomas, Gaskin, and Herriot, 1979)

This series has been designed for use with children in the early stages of communication (originally, limited-ability youngsters) and is concerned with processes of 'understanding, speaking and feedback'. The material consists of three boxes of card drawings, vividly coloured, introducing a central character, Jim, and his family, in various situations. Accompanying booklets give general suggestions for use. In teaching *understanding* a child might be asked to point to the card which shows a boy painting a door; cards are used as a basis for *speaking*: 'What's this? This is a ...'; whilst *feedback* involves discussion of the feelings and reactions of characters depicted on the cards. Each boxed set presents situations, and therefore teaching points, of increasing complexity; for example, in a later series the child may be asked 'Show me where dad *is going to* shave.' Two assumptions underpin the series: firstly, that children who fail to learn need deliberate exposure to carefully graded language teaching; secondly, that material should be simple, bright, and relevant. Many teachers have found the material useful, simply because it provides a context for flexible teaching.

Game Oriented Activities for Learning, levels 1 and 2 (Karnes, 1977)

GOAL is an American programme designed for children with limited ability, speech and language difficulties, or English as a second language. Level 1 is for children aged three to five years, level 2 for children of school age. GOAL uses a game strategy to foster a wide range of language processes, acquire new concepts and ideas, relate new to prior information, draw conclusions, communicate facts to others, and enhance creative and problem-solving abilities. The clinical model of the Illinois Test of Psycholinguistic Abilities is used as the theoretical framework for developing the lesson plans of GOAL. Language teaching is broken down into the 10 areas of ITPA and ideas are prescribed for each, intended for use in daily 30-minute sessions with small groups. For example, in developing *auditory association*, level 1 asks children to name three items that belong to a mother, father, brother, sister, and baby. At level 2 children are asked to think of the workers associated with words such as 'menu', 'barn', or 'patient'. Examples which foster *manual expression* include, at level 1, pretending to put on articles of clothing, such as pants or socks. At level 2, children mirror a set of actions, such as raising an arm or leg, performed by a partner. Ideas for facilitating *visual closure* comprise, at level 1, recognising fruits which have been cut into slices; whilst at level 2, children identify traffic signs from their shapes. Lastly, as examples of *auditory memory*, suggestions include, for younger children, remembering and performing a two-item set of directions, such as 'shut the door, then wiggle.' For older children, sequences of drum beats are reproduced as 'rhythm messages'. Teachers find the abundance of game activities to be a useful classroom resource which can be used flexibly and selectively. The material suffers from the same criticisms generally applied to the use of ITPA: uncertainty as to whether working on cognitive skills improves language as a direct consequence. Nevertheless, the material can be used to provide enjoyable activities, which indirectly create an interactive learning context.

Direct Instructional Systems to Arithmetic and Reading: Language 1 (Engelmann and Osborn, 1976)

DISTAR is one of a number of 'direct instruction' programmes which have emanated from the United States. The distinctive aspect of DISTAR is not the materials which make up the programmes, but the set of teaching principles which underlie them. The authors have aimed at designing a faultless learning environment for the efficient teaching of skills, which then generalise to other settings. DISTAR is for use with 'special needs' children in general, including hearing-impaired, from nursery age onwards. Teaching is essentially in small groups of five to ten children for daily 30-minute sessions, so some organisational planning is required. The subject matter of each lesson is broken down into small, discrete tasks, which are presented in a rigid and repetitive way. The teacher's actions and words are stipulated, even to defining the manner of pointing at picture materials. The teacher works through each task by demonstrating the correct procedure, leading the children by question and answer through the exercise, demanding individual responses to test understanding, reinforcing target responses with praise, correcting mistakes, and then repeating the whole task. It has been calculated that every child answers between two and three hundred questions in the course of a 30-minute lesson.

The main DISTAR language materials consist of five teacher presentation books of 160 lessons, beginning with object identification. For example, children are shown a picture of a bottle and taken through a series of questions with prescribed instructions and acceptable responses: 'Is this a fish? ... Say the whole thing with me. ... This is *not* a fish.' An important aspect is that children are not simply taught the correct labels, they are also introduced to concept boundaries: examples which are not covered by the target vocabulary, and which therefore help the child to use words appropriately in other contexts. DISTAR moves through aspects of language such as prepositions, pronouns, verbs and their tenses; question words, such as 'who', 'what', 'where'; comparatives, such as 'same', 'different'; temporal sequence, for example, 'before', 'after'; category functions, such as animals or containers; leading to problem solving and abstract concepts. DISTAR teaches continuously to criteria, with frequent probes to check what the child has retained and to determine choice of objectives for future teaching.

The programmes have been evaluated by teachers in special education with generally favourable reactions. There is evidence that children gain in confidence, concentration and language skills through its use. Some teachers feel the materials are poorly illustrated and lack interest value. Others object to the rigid drills and massed practice which have to be repeated in a teaching framework where the child is mainly responding to questions. The 'faultless' teaching environment described by the authors of DISTAR, with its ordered sequence of learning steps, may be reassuring to teachers who are uncertain how to approach children with severe language delays, or what to teach next. However, much of what we have said in the earlier chapters of this book about children's functional discovery of language, in shared, purposeful contexts, is difficult to reconcile with the DISTAR teaching model.

Living Language (Locke, 1985)

This is a remedial teaching programme produced in the United Kingdom for children from pre-school to 16 years of age who are failing to learn to speak spontaneously. Locke's argument is that, for language-delayed children, the school is often a poor language-learning environment compared with the adult–child interactive contexts found at home. The author's scheme was designed to foster the flow of language by encouraging adult responsiveness, providing experiences built around children's interests, and exposing children to a redundancy of input through frequent repetition. Teaching sessions are seen as supplementary to reinforcement of the language already used in school. In one sense 'Living Language' can be viewed as a syllabus of appropriate teaching content, together with a set of strategies for the teacher.

The material itself consists of a handbook and three manuals covering areas of *Pre-Language*, *First Words* and *Putting Words Together*. Teacher strategies are behavioural in the main, based on clear target setting within a framework of sequenced objectives; but more recent ideas regarding the rooting of language use in day-to-day events are integrated into the scheme. The first vocabulary items to be taught include body parts, clothes, toys, vehicles, people, and action verbs such as 'hit', 'walk', 'cut', 'cry', and 'push'. The syllabus of language activities includes personal feelings, eating and drinking, the playground, bedtime, shops and towns, people and their bodies, time, the weather, properties and relationships; together with object qualities like colour, texture, sound, shape, and movement. Little evaluation of the scheme has been carried out as yet, but its adaptable, pragmatic approach may appeal to many teachers who resist the overprescriptive and limiting methods of other programmes.

Derbyshire Language Scheme (Knowles and Masidlover, 1982)

The DLS was developed by a speech therapist and an educational psychologist in a special school setting for children with a range of learning difficulties and with delayed language skills. Unlike many programmes, the DLS is not a schedule of lessons to be carried out in a set sequence. It is a collection of activities aimed at fostering specific language skills derived from practical experience. Two aspects of the DLS should be highlighted: firstly, teaching strategies embrace current thinking, for example, on the importance of adult–child interaction in language development. Secondly, activities chosen by the teacher are closely linked, in an ongoing way, with a careful system of observation and assessment. The DLS enables teachers to assess a child's understanding and use of language according to a normal developmental framework, up to the age of about four and a half years.

The scheme is implemented using a 'Rapid Screening Test' which guides the teacher to the appropriate level of a 'Detailed Test of Comprehension'. This has three main sections: basic vocabulary, and single element sentences; two- to four-word stages; and levels 5 to 10 which move through a wide range of grammatical aspects such as use of different tenses, prepositions, negatives, pronouns, and questions. A play context is also provided for obtaining a sample of the child's expressive language. The scheme gives very detailed outlines of the toy materials to be used at each stage level based on the Reynell (1969) model, and includes a book of picture materials which help the examiner to decide on the child's functional control of grammatical structures of different kinds and at different levels. Information on each child's performance on the 'Detailed Test of Comprehension' is recorded on a score sheet and transferred to an 'Assessment Summary and Progress Record'. The assessment coding is cross-referenced to teaching activities in the teacher's manual. So, at every level of the scheme, the examiner has immediate access to ideas for remediating a specific aspect of language.

Unlike the majority of the programmes reviewed in this chapter, the DLS escapes criticism on several fronts. In the first place, the child is not seen as a passive recipient of language training, but is involved actively in spontaneous interactions. For example, a key teaching strategy is role-reversal in which the child takes control of the activity, by giving commands and asking questions of the adult. This has been found to be highly motivating to most children, providing them with a demonstration of the power speech has to affect others, whilst also avoiding the pitfalls described by Wood and Wood (1984), whereby children with limited language tend to be subject to an increase in teacher-control and less nurturing styles of interaction. In the second place, DLS avoids focussing on the form of correct language. The emphasis, instead, lies with the 'eliciting context'. For example, a tea-party game might be chosen to encourage 'more plus a noun', where the language arises naturally out of the play situation. Finally, besides paying attention to the social processes of language use, DLS also shows some awareness of the cognitive aspects of language, such as familiarity with real objects, symbolic play and more abstract picture awareness. It does not cover the latter so well as the scheme devised by Cooper, Moodley and Reynell (1978) but is much richer in suggestions for the teacher. The major attraction of the DLS, to those who have learned how to use it, is the diversity of play opportunities and teaching activities given in the teacher's manual.

Although the underlying ideas of the DLS are straightforward, the scheme is technically difficult to master and is not readily digestible without the help of a trained tutor. It is very revealing that having been trained to use the DLS, many teachers dispense with the manuals and learn more from *doing* the scheme, rather than reading the over-wrought and complex guidelines. One common complaint is that the expressive scale is much less easy to use than the receptive, and depends on length rather than sophistication of syntax. Whilst the scheme claims to cover language used and understood by normal children up to four and a half years of age, the majority of the structures covered are within the age range one and a half to two and a half years and later stages are too narrow. Teachers put up with the tribulations of the presentation and format because the DLS provides extremely useful suggestions for play opportunities, materials, teaching objectives and strategies, for use with small groups, particularly in the early stages of language work.

COMPUTER-ASSISTED LEARNING

Before long most primary and secondary schools will have access to microcomputers and this survey of teaching packages would be incomplete without some reference to the array of software which is commercially available. At first sight, computer programs designed for children with special needs in speech and language appear to have some marked advantages. Material is presented visually to the child and has the potential for overcoming many of the obstacles to communication which characterise other oral language-learning contexts. Most children find microcomputers stimulating and highly-motivating; good programs present individually paced learning steps controlled by the child; and there is immediate feedback to responses. These aspects fulfil some of the conditions for learning set down by Gagné and discussed in chapter 3.

Language software can be described in terms of four categories (Rushby, 1979). *Instructional* software requires the child to master concepts in the program. Practice can be given in the correct use of verbs, adverbs, prepositions, and past tenses, supported by graphics. A program designed to teach the vocabulary of shapes exposes words along with the corresponding shape, such as a hexagon. When the child punches the correct word into the keyboard, a musical or visual treat is given on the screen as a reward. Several programs have been designed to teach receptive vocabulary, such as names of animals, body parts, clothing, utensils, food, toys, and vehicles. Picture pairs are presented and the child asked to make a selection: 'Show me the fork.' In another example, opposite pairs are presented, such as empty/full. A glass appears and is filled with juice by pressing an arrow key. Activating another arrow key empties the glass. A homonym program provides a highlighted word in the context of a sentence and the child has to find substitutes for the word. Subskills of reading, such as phonic blends, can be taught in step-by-step fashion. Children may be asked to recognise sound and letter correspondences, or to identify phonic blends. Spelling games present words which then have to be reproduced by the child. Incorrect entries are dealt with, in one example, by a 'gremlin' digging out the wrong letters and burying them in a hole; sadly, correct entries are not so spectacularly rewarded.

In a second kind of *revelatory* program, the child gradually discovers linked pieces of information in the subject material. In some typical examples, children explore caves, use clues to find a dragon's magical teeth, search for Egyptian tombs, and find the way out of a haunted waxworks. The third category of software is *conjectural*. Here children test out ideas and hypotheses within the program. An invisible ink task requires the child to uncover hidden words by guessing from the surrounding context and picture clues. A shipwreck program sets the problem of how to build a boat to escape from an island, with a sequence of branching routines which respond to the child's queries. Some software uses a variation of the 'cloze' technique, whereby sentences are presented to the child with gaps for completion, testing the child's understanding and awareness of grammatical constraints.

A fourth category of software is described as *emancipatory* since traditional teaching techniques are enhanced. In one program a child's free written work is simply scanned for spelling mistakes. A computerised thesaurus has been devised which suggests alternative words to those given by the child in composing a sentence. In other text-creation programs, children produce stories from their own personal word stores, whilst text-editing facilities allow children to see and amend their sentences before they are printed out. Some programs animate written commands and illustrate concepts entered into the keyboard by the child. In one example, sentences such as 'The boy jumps', 'The cats dance', 'The dog walks' are animated on the screen, but the vocabulary and sentence types are limited. A fresh approach to familiar nursery rhymes has been produced by one software designer. In a 'Three Bears' package, the child punches in directions for progressing through the story, such as 'G' for Goldilocks, 'S' for stirring the porridge, and 'J' for jumping on the bed. The story proceeds according to the choices selected by the children and there is opportunity for role play, with a number of children taking a part in the story. A range of alternative keyboards and storyboards are now available, some with words, symbols, or pictures, others with scenarios which can be animated, the point being to give the child the experience of watching language forms come to life.

Computer-assisted approaches to language intervention are not, however, a panacea. There are serious problems in designing software for young children where the language content to be taught is often far less complex than the task instructions. Demands made on the child in understanding objects and concepts graphically represented, in manipulating a keyboard and indicating selections, may also be underestimated. However, the major criticism of computer intervention is inherent in all direct teaching approaches, and this is an issue which is addressed more fully in chapter 5.

In all natural language-learning contexts, language is discovered by the child in shared interactive contexts where the focus is upon communication. Despite the potential of computers for arousing curiosity, self-pacing, and increased motivation, the majority of programs foster a respondent, decontextualized style of language behaviour in which the child is a passive recipient of software prompts and demands. It is questionable just how much language rehearsed in this non-interactive way generalises to other, more genuine communication contexts. It could be claimed that the language learned by the child is limited in scope, stereotypic and lacking in social function. However, it is possible to use microcomputers as a means of establishing a social context for learning, where the child and adult interact around the program content (Miller and Marriner, 1986). So, for example, text-editing software and story-boards provide an opportunity for joint composition between child and adult, in which the computer supports the topic of conversation.

In summary, teachers should be aware of the range of assessment materials and teaching schemes which are currently available for children with language difficulties. Test materials must be used selectively, with a steady eye on the purpose of assessment and the nature of the information required. It is clear that tests which summarise a child's developmental level in an area of language may be useful in providing an overall picture of a child for others, or in demonstrating progress over time. However, teachers may require more specific information, such as the contrast between a child's phonetic maturity and the level of symbolic play, and tests should be selected accordingly. Tests provide supportive information and help to build up a profile of a child, but cannot be expected to give penetrating insights. They may well allow the teacher to devise a set of objectives within the normal developmental framework. Similarly, commercial materials may provide a useful source of ideas for the teacher to develop, particularly when the focus of interventions is on 'eliciting contexts', rather than on dispensing language bit-by-bit from a package, without regard to the social and interactive functions of natural language learning contexts. Both language tests and language schemes alter the nature of the communication experience for the adult and child, and that may be unhelpful.

—5

Language intervention

*There is no set of rules of how to talk to a child that can even approach
what you unconsciously know.*

(Brown, 1977, page 26)

Brown is responding above to the question 'How can a child's
learning of language be facilitated?' In thinking of the ways in which
teachers can help children communicate we have, like Brown, taken
as our starting point the skills and strategies of the natural and
spontaneous parent. A great deal of what we have to say is either an
enhancement or clarification of what adults normally do. We do not
believe that language can be dispensed to children, or taught as a
subject set apart from the rest of the child's learning experience.
When teachers ask what they need to do differently should a child
have communication problems, the simple answer is *to communicate*.
In Brown's terms (1977, page 12), that means 'to understand and to
be understood'. When conditions for communication are right, the
child's active impetus for language learning will be harnessed.
Make communication purposeful and meaningful and the child will
be motivated to discover language through using it. In other words,
the adult stimulates and facilitates language interaction, but it is the
child's task to piece together the rules of the game.

The underlying philosophy of this approach is that children's
communication difficulties are best understood by observing how
children use language in the different environments in which they
live, play, and learn. Instead of seeing language difficulties as
residing wholly within the child, attention is focussed on the
patterns of interaction between child and others. In planning
language intervention we shall be emphasising factors in the adult's
style of behaviour, the physical organisation of the school,
co-ordination of support agencies and resources, and aspects
of the curriculum. These are the major variables which teachers
can control. As we saw in chapter 3, a diversity of factors
influence the child's potential for learning, such as intact senses,
physical and intellectual skills, and a nurturing family environment.
Most, if not all, of these variables are *outside* the teachers' control. It
follows that by optimising conditions for learning and developing

strategies for language interaction to take place, the effort invested is much more likely to be repaid. Where the learning context is given a low order of priority in face of more obvious learning obstacles, such as a severe hearing loss, or the limited ability customarily associated with Down's syndrome, then we may be guilty of exacerbating a child's difficulties by providing less-than-nurturing opportunities in which the child can progress.

The term 'naturalistic' has sometimes been applied to the approach we recommend (Müller, 1984). In order to apply such an approach we have to be absolutely clear about the natural circumstances in which spontaneous language interaction takes place. One central process we shall be discussing concerns the strategies for conversation adopted by adults. Adjustments to adult speech in contexts of meaningful activity provide clear evidence from which children can learn. The view that language cannot be taught directly, or in isolation, but reflects the sharing of experience, should not imply that we can be hazy in our thinking about the objectives of our teaching. The starting point must always be a careful consideration of where the child is in terms of the skills already mastered, and what we hope the child will achieve. The next step is to use the teaching objectives which have been set, in order to plan appropriate learning opportunities. Whether, in fact, the teaching experience is a fostering and helpful one for the child concerned, can only be gauged by monitoring whether the objectives are achieved over time.

The major differences between the approach advocated here and other kinds of intervention are ones of focus and of control. The present focus lies on the communication context: the social situations in which language arises, what it means to the participants, the intentions realised through using it, and the patterns of interaction between children and adults which enhance language development. Language behaviour is spontaneous in the sense that contributions are made freely, without external control. Other approaches, such as behaviour therapy (see review by Müller, 1980), have been based on techniques derived from learning theory, usually applied in a clinical setting, in which language is deliberately controlled by a therapist. Responses such as looking behaviour, sounds or words may be elicited from the child and then reinforced in some way, perhaps by rewarding the child with food or praise. The focus of attention is on the form, or content, of what the child says, rather than the social interaction between the people involved.

Direct teaching techniques, where the child is a passive participant in language exercises set by a teacher or therapist, are usually justified on the grounds that a child has already failed to learn in more 'natural' contexts. Several points need to be made here, without wishing to be didactic, so that teachers can make informed choices about the way they work. Firstly, few nursery or school environments may *actually* provide the richness of language interaction employed by children at home, although they may claim to be 'natural'. Schools, therefore, can be helped towards more nurturing styles of interaction. Secondly, individualised training of specific language skills has its pitfalls. A great deal of time is usually required to improve performance across what is usually a very narrow range of language forms. The most fundamental criticism, however, is that language learnt during training may not be used spontaneously by the child in other settings, and the function of language in the child's social world may be ignored. (For an elaboration of these points, see Rutter, 1980.) As we said earlier in relation to language 'kits' and programmes, highly structured interventions alter the nature of the linguistic and social environment in ways which may be unhelpful to language learning.

Those who have been developing 'behavioural' methods of teaching have, in fact, moved on from individual training to a far more ecological approach which takes into account relationships between the child and the environment necessary for language development. 'Behavioural' and 'natural' styles are not necessarily incompatible. In a recent paper by Rogers-Warren, Warren, and Baer (1983) 'ideal' environments for language learning are described, which incorporate elements of normal interactive settings, together with behavioural principles, such as feedback and reinforcement. For those who feel strongly that children need deliberate exposure to specific items of language, there is no reason why language lessons should not be designed to strengthen the learning from less formal settings. A short period could be set aside for this kind of practice session as an adjunct to the child's day-to-day language experience. For the teacher working within a mainstream school setting, some thought needs to be given to what is practicable and appropriate, as well as theoretically plausible. The strategies for intervention which follow are based, to a greater or lesser degree, on the belief that language is learned through complex interactive processes involving children and adults, as they live, play and learn together.

SUPPORT SYSTEMS AND INTEGRATION

Enthusiasm for helping children with communication needs within mainstream settings stems from the growing awareness of the importance of context on the way in which language is used and understood. Children make communication demands on each other and are often at their most animated in the company of peers. We have suggested that informal social situations, with no explicit direction or control, are very important in language learning. Children learn just as much by talking to others about what they are doing, whether in playing pinball, at home over the dinner table, in the changing room, or in the snack bar, as they do in formal teaching periods. However, the idea behind flexible support systems for children is to help achieve the right kind of balance between peer-group exposure and more individualised time with an adult. All teachers are aware that children with special needs who are left entirely unsupported, both in informal settings and in teaching contexts, may be overwhelmed by the demands they have to face and can switch off completely. Naturally, then, the very first questions which many teachers ask in relation to children with communication difficulties in the mainstream school, are to do with resources. The most important of all resources in schools are human: the number of pairs of adult hands to the wheel.

The overall responsibility for a special needs child in an ordinary classroom should be taken by the class teacher. It is, however, important for teachers to know what kind of specialist advice is available, whether a child will be given any supportive help, and how a programme of intervention is to be planned, co-ordinated and shared between the adults involved. Every child's needs should be appraised carefully and individually, in line with the recent philosophy that we should try to fit arrangements flexibly to children, rather than children to schools. Whatever provision is recommended, professional advisers must take into account a number of factors together with the needs of the child. These include the availability of resources within a particular school, and it is to these that attention is turned first of all. Occasionally, a school will already have additional help, such as a classroom assistant, organised to meet the special needs identified in other children. It may be possible to extend and sustain this extra help when a new child is identified. In some local authorities, support teams, including language and remedial teaching specialists, are normally available to schools, to be drawn in to help children on a regular basis, as and when appropriate. Speech therapists are available in some areas to give advice in schools, help plan a suitable programme with a teacher, and, occasionally, to work with an individual child in the school setting. The multi-professional team involved with children who experience communication difficulties will address the question: 'Can this particular child's needs be met within the resources normally available to this particular school?' If not, the formal statutory procedures under the 1981 Act are initiated to ascertain exactly what the child's needs are and how they might be met.

In some local education authorities it is the practice to collect children together in one resourced mainstream school, where additional language specialists, or a speech therapist, are available to help. Arrangements are often flexible, depending on the needs of the child. Some children are able to participate for the majority of the time in ordinary classes, with a specialist teacher supporting the work in mainstream education by giving additional help to supplement information presented in class, reinforce key concepts, check understanding, and prepare the child for future lessons. As we have said, the responsibility for what is taught in a mainstream class must be with the class teacher. But, if a child is going to spend time out of class for supportive help and if more than one adult is going to be involved, then teachers must work carefully together. Detailed forward planning is perhaps the most difficult, although potentially most valuable, groundwork for supporting children with special needs in mainstream classes. We shall be returning to this idea again when we consider curricular planning in more detail.

CLASSROOM MANAGEMENT

Extra adult bodies in the classroom has been called the key to integration (Thomas, 1985). Since talk with adults appears to be the fundamental language-learning encounter, proper management of adult resources in the mainstream has to be considered. Achieving additional classroom help is not an end in itself and a great deal of thought has to be given to how such a resource can be managed effectively. Extra adult help may come from parents, ancillary helpers, specialist teachers, or perhaps speech therapists. But unless tasks and roles are clearly defined, there will be confusion as to who is doing what and with whom.

A number of distinct roles can be described. The class teacher may wish to act as overall manager, organising space, time, and materials for the larger group, or groups, of children in the class, taking charge of discipline, together with rules about noise and movement. The manager's job might include presenting tasks and activities to the class, prompting children to be busy, moving around the group to give minimal attention to individuals, such as brief help and praise. Thomas (1985) suggests that one important aspect of a teacher's role is to maintain *flow* through a session, keeping children engaged on task, with a sense of purpose and impetus. An extra adult might help sustain flow by dealing with interruptions. This adult could move quickly from child to child, dealing with questions, providing information and feedback, and discussing the point of the enquiry. At another level the adult may be assigned to work with three or four individual children for set periods of, say, 15 minutes each. The individual helper's role might include preparing or using special materials, drawing the child's attention to the task in hand, checking understanding, organising the sequence of learning steps, helping the child to reflect, extract concepts, relate one idea to another, and make judgements, motivating the child and providing the kind of intensive conversational interaction which foster what Tizard and Hughes (1984) have called 'passages of intellectual search'.

Classroom management enables adults to share a depth and intensity of responsiveness to children, which may characterise the learning context of the home more frequently than that of the school. We have already mentioned the work of Gagné (1977) who also has a lot to say about the conditions which surround learning. Extra adults in class can fulfil some important requirements for effective learning, including giving opportunities for frequent regular practice of a skill in a situation of rapid feedback and praise; helping children to discover and reinforce concepts by having many examples to consider; cueing the children by supplying the right word to fix their experience; and guiding the children's thinking to the point where they uncover solutions for themselves.

In a very useful paper, Anderson, Evertson and Emmer (1980) have listed specific adult behaviours which contribute to better classroom management, and these are particularly important for children with communication needs, whatever class role the adult has adopted. A sense of purpose is established by adults who help children to pace their activities within the time available, giving regular and systematic feedback, and isolating the main features of the task. Better managers give clear expectations about behaviour, such as how (and how not) to ask for help, address a teacher, sit on a rug, or knock on a door. They do not assume that children can follow instructions without checking, and very specific feedback is given: 'Well done for remembering that only two people at a time are to use the guillotine.' Most importantly, better managers start and stop activities very clearly, giving warnings before any topic changes. Strategies for gaining children's attention are well worked out, such as arranging desks so that children face a point where attention is most often focussed; moderating voice; beginning with 'settling-in' activities before introducing more demanding work; presenting one task at a time, rather than simultaneously; and requiring active attention when important information is given by, for example, asking children to close their books whilst listening.

LANGUAGE UNITS

There are some children, usually those with more severe communication difficulties, whose needs cannot be met entirely by support in the mainstream. These may be children who find difficulties in learning, even with extra help, in larger group situations. Such children may only feel comfortable in a more protected, secure environment with a predictable framework and routine of events, and where the teacher has time to make close relationships with all the members of the group. Again, this is a question of balance: the right mix of peer-group exposure and more individualised adult help.

Some local authorities have already resourced mainstream schools at the primary level, with units for children with speech and language difficulties, staffed by specialist language teachers and speech therapists who work closely together. Units are an important part of the continuum of provision for children with special needs (see table 5.1) and work most effectively when there is flexibility. Some children may need to spend the larger proportion of the school day with the specialist teacher in the unit, covering basic skills and formal aspects of the curriculum, such as mathematics. Integration into larger mainstream groups may need to be broached gradually, starting with practically-orientated subjects, or areas where a child may already show confidence and skill, such as games, cookery, dance, pottery, gymnastics. There will be very few children who cannot enjoy some of the play and social opportunities on offer in school, even though the academic core is to be found in the unit. As we have said, some of the most purposeful communication contexts, in which children make demands on each other, around subjects of vital interest to the participants, are found at mealtimes, during break, in after-school clubs and playground games, and in all the interest groups which surround school. Some would argue that the success of a child's integration programme can be measured by how far the child shares the 'real' community of the school – being included in pantomime trips, excursions, visits, and sports teams, taking part in fund-raising days and concerts, and presenting assemblies.

In a unit setting, language resources can be gathered and expertise developed, whilst the whole can be a local centre for advice and materials. Children have the advantage of more frequent

Table 5.1 *A continuum of provision for children with speech and language difficulties*

Placement in a mainstream class – occasional monitoring and help from language specialist or speech therapist.

Mainstream class with additional help in some subject areas from language support teacher, remedial specialist, plus speech therapy.

Ordinary class with tutorial help: child is withdrawn for extra help by a specialist teacher, or teacher's assistant on a daily or weekly basis across a range of subjects, with speech therapy.

Resource unit in a mainstream school: special class with varying degrees of integration in ordinary groups. Usually combined with more intensive language activities and speech therapy.

Special school as a base with part-time integration into ordinary classes and speech therapy input.

Full-time special school with intensive specialised teaching and speech therapy.

and intense contact with specialist teachers and therapists, who are able to plan more thoroughly to meet a child's individual profile of needs. A unit may provide a sense of continuity and act as a refuge for children who find the stresses and changes of a mainstream school daunting. There is time to gear work specifically towards helping a child's communication difficulties in a wide range of curriculum areas and to co-ordinate this appropriately with experiences in mainstream. In some language units, 'reverse' integration is practised whereby children from ordinary class groups join in selected unit activities. If 'unit' children are to feel an integral part of the school community, physical location in the main body of the school, as opposed to a 'terrapin' or portable classroom at the bottom of the playground, is important. So too, shared playtimes, lunchbreaks, starting and finishing points, with no essential differences in the framework of the school day, are important.

SPECIAL SCHOOL

At the far end of the range of provision available for children with speech and language difficulties given in table 5.1, special school may be recommended on a part or full-time basis. Special schools are usually set up with high adult–child ratios and staff who are trained and interested in working with children who have exceptional difficulties. There are very few children who require this kind of specialised environment solely because of their communication needs. Sometimes a special school is recommended when the child has a combination of severe special needs, including language. The handful of schools which cater for speech and language difficulties are residential in the main. The idea behind such a school placement is that the whole living, playing, and learning environment is designed to help the child communicate. Sometimes a child may have failed to learn in an ordinary school or unit situation, before a special school is recommended. It may be more acceptable to parents for a child to be placed away from home at the secondary stage, when the demands of school, both socially and academically, are greater and the child is more mature. On the other hand children who go at an earlier age for intensive special school help can be expected to make more progress than older ones, with the prospect of returning to mainstream. Always, the balance of benefits for the child in a specialised environment has to be weighed against the disadvantages, such as distance from the family, loss of contact with local children and a more restricted educational curriculum.

One clear example of a situation in which a special school might be recommended is where a child has such limited understanding of language and such poor expressive skills, that it is impossible for the child to establish friendships, to take part in group work and to participate in any meaningful way in an ordinary school community. An alternative means of communication, such as a sign language, may be suggested as a support to speech. The Paget–Gorman sign system, to take an example, is made up of series of hand shapes and movements which reflect the spoken grammatical structure of English and can be used to illustrate visually what the speaker is saying. It is usually felt that if a child's needs are so special as to warrant an esoteric means of communication, then these needs are probably best met in a special school where the whole body of teaching and ancillary staff are able to use the system and are convinced of its effectiveness. This is not to say that signing as a support to spoken language will never be encountered in resourced mainstream schools. However, there are likely to be severe restrictions on the social and linguistic interactions enjoyed by children in a context where only a minority are taught how to sign.

THE LISTENING ENVIRONMENT

In a good local education authority there will be a range of facilities for helping children, a flexible variety of resources which can be adapted to meet the individual circumstances of the child. One factor, common to all environments in which children with speech and language difficulties are helped, concerns acoustic conditions. In the early stages, particularly, the teacher's efforts will be directed towards attention control and listening skills. Children do not attend or listen effectively in noisy, reverberant conditions replete with distracting sounds. For the child with a known hearing difficulty, even if this is a mild, fluctuating conductive loss, the listening environment should be sympathetic. We have suggested that one important function of language is to help mediate and shape the child's learning experience. It follows that all children with a delay or specific difficulty in acquiring language will be less able to deal with incoming information, with their auditory and perceptual experiences. Hence, a basic starter is to provide good listening conditions, at least for some of the child's day.

There are several aspects to consider. Firstly, keeping unwanted noise out. Children are less likely to listen in a room which is regularly invaded by the noise of cars and lorries from a busy road, an upstairs workshop, the clattering of feet from a busy corridor, a gymnasium, music room, or dance studio, and where there is no door to close on outside activities. The second consideration is the reduction of noise within a room. Hard floors, concrete posts, high ceilings, and cladded walls reverberate sound and make for listening difficulties. Soft furnishings, carpeted areas, rubber boots on chairs, soft table tops, cork-tiled walls, curtained windows, all reduce reverberant noise. Children will generally listen more attentively to each other, to a story, or to the teacher, in conditions away from noise sources such as a well-used sink area, passageway or store cupboard. In some situations teachers deliberately reduce other kinds of distractions, in order to enhance the child's focus of attention. Children with very fleeting attention span may prefer to work on their own or in small groups in 'booths': small partitioned areas. The child faces away from the main activities of the room and there are fewer visual distractions because the walls of the booth are bare and simply obscure the child's immediate visual field. Whilst it may rarely be necessary to go to lengths such as these, many school contexts are extremely noisy, distracting places. Large, open-plan, busy classrooms may generate a lot of noise and a plethora of distractions which make it even more difficult for the child with a speech or language problem to learn.

TEACHING OBJECTIVES

In chapter 1 we identified some of the central concerns shared by all schools, for all children, with and without special needs. For example, a general aim of most teachers is to help children to achieve independence, to think clearly, to describe and then categorise events, to extract concepts as part of a growing understanding of the world, and to be capable of predicting a likely course of events. Eventually, teaching goals will embrace a knowledge of written language as well as the intellectual functions served by spoken language. It is not easy to translate the general aims of teaching into specific learning objectives for an individual child. Stated in a general way, it may not always be clear when a particular child has reached an important educational goal: at what point, for example, can we be sure a child has become 'an independent thinker'? For this reason, it may be helpful to set down teaching objectives in a more precise form for each child. We may need to spell out the specific skills or patterns of behaviour we intend a child to have mastered by the end of the teaching process. A number of authors working with children who experience global learning difficulties (Ainscow and Tweddle, 1979), or who have language difficulties (White and East, 1981), suggest that effective teaching begins with a clear statement of what the child needs to learn. Having decided what to teach, thought can then be given to teaching method and how best to organise the child's learning experience within the resources available. It is at this point that the child's profile of educational objectives must be considered in relation to the school curriculum – an issue we shall be looking at subsequently.

There are several good reasons to set down a clear profile of teaching objectives. In the first place, there may be many professionals, other than teachers, involved with the child and objectives should be agreed upon through discussion so that the targets to aim for are clear to all concerned. Secondly, identification of what it is hoped the child will learn provides a framework for evaluating progress over time. Continual assessment of a child's achievements must have clear reference points, which an individual learning programme provides. Although we have deliberately emphasised informal, natural and active processes of language learning (as opposed to direct, structured teaching) this does not imply that we can be equivocal or hazy in our teaching objectives.

Where to begin? All good teaching, at all stages of schooling, starts from where the learner is. Careful assessment, taking into account the insights of parents, psychologist, speech therapist, doctor, and teachers, should reveal the developmental level of the child. We need to establish what the child can and cannot do in different skill areas, and what needs to be tackled next. In a number of aspects of language development we can highlight appropriate skills for a child of a given age. In chapter 2 we described various aspects of normal language acquisition and the ordinary sequence of stages through which language unfolds. A knowledge of the natural learning steps which all children take enables us to locate an individual's current achievements and to plan realistic and developmentally appropriate teaching targets. The complementary role of more formal, or commercially available materials in the assessment and remediation process, has been discussed in chapter 4. In specifying teaching objectives, we must take account of each child's pace of learning, since some children require rather smaller learning steps than others, with a shorter distance between them. This kind of detailed statement of a child's learning needs may appear to be a laborious exercise. However, we will never know whether a child has reached a teaching target, unless we are clear about what we are aiming at in the first place. We give below some thoroughly worked examples of teaching objectives for individual children, each involving a description of the child, teaching objectives, and adult strategies.

Teaching objectives for a pre-school child with developmental language delay

Description of child

> *Robert at three and a half years has about ten recognisable words; is reluctant to speak even in relaxed, familiar settings; communicates largely by gesture, or relies on smiles and nods. His play is age-appropriate but he has a fleeting attention and poor fine motor control; for example, he is a very messy drinker, particularly with a straw. He is reluctant to separate from his mother, to approach others, or join in a story group, and tends to be silent but watchful. He needs help to establish relationships, develop joint play, explore his environment, sustain attention, and build up communication skills.*

Teaching objectives

- Sustain eye-contact with speaker
- Separate confidently from parent
- Join in play activity with one adult or child
- Hold attention on task or listening to a story for a five-minute period
- Use finger and thumb pincer grip to pick up small objects
- Hold scissors, pencil, brush correctly
- Take turns in games with another child
- Sort objects according to colour, shape, size
- Vocalise during play
- Join in pretend play with small group
- Participate in group rhymes, songs, and jingles
- Locate and refer to everyday objects, people, and activities by name

- Indicate needs through words as well as gestures
- Respond appropriately to simple verbal cues, directions, and questions, such as a two-element instruction
- Initiate interaction by approaching adult or child with a request for materials and toys
- Request vocabulary for familiar items and events
- Trace over model words, copy name accurately
- Associate a word with a picture to attempt a guess

Adult strategies

- Provide a secure and accepting environment with familiar routines, e.g. milk and biscuit – 'yes please', 'thank you'
- Accompany own activity with talk
- Restrict number of adults in contact with child and introduce him to other children with adult present, initially
- Praise 'on-task' behaviour
- Discuss least obtrusive way of parent leaving child in nursery, record progress in home–school book
- Provide a range of opportunities for fine manipulative play, such as cutting, pasting, threading, folding, sewing, drawing, painting, clay or plasticine modelling
- Set up games, joint tasks, pretend play where child has opportunities for turn-taking
- Involve children in a story by providing pictures of main characters, acting out the story using handpuppets, toys or storyboard, make sound effects
- Provide toy animals, dolls, puppets, vehicles, play people and a variety of construction materials, and both give and encourage commentary on activity
- Encourage small group role play in Wendy House, shop setting, office, cafe, tent, using dressing-up clothes such as shoes, hats, wigs, noses
- Give opportunities for small group singing, clapping and action songs in which children can join, such as 'I can hammer ... ', 'If you're happy and you know it ... '
- Use a consistent vocabulary for toilet, playtime, drink, familiar events, and people
- Respond to child's utterances with sentences which expand and clarify meaning, including words which the child has used
- Tie activities and events to pictures, stories and written words

Teaching objectives for a six-year-old child with immature phonology

Description of child

> Susan is often unintelligible to everyone except her immediate family who understand her in the context of their home environment and interpret her speech for others. She has little rhythmic sense and is unable to hear rhyming words, although hearing is normal. Susan is reticent at asking questions and has strategies for avoiding language interaction, such as lowering head and gaze. There is no apparent difficulty with verbal comprehension (age-appropriate levels on British Picture Vocabulary Scale and Reynell Receptive Language Scale). A significant aspect is her loss of confidence and negative anticipation. She has just begun to recognise simple sight words and copy words from a model.

Teaching objectives

- Be confident enough to request help, materials or services from an adult, using gestures and words
- Respond appropriately to body language and non-verbal signals
- Have a reliable vocabulary of clearly articulated words, such as 'b' words like ball, bike, boy
- To look at person attempting to gain her attention
- Follow conversation by watching other speakers
- Initiate spoken interactions with other children in play
- Recount the sequence of events in a familiar story using picture cues
- Talk about immediate experiences, use language to direct and organise activities
- Repeat a drum rhythm, clap a regular accent in a rhyme or piece of music, march in time to music
- Role-play telephone conversations or ask for items in a shop
- Construct stories using a 'Breakthrough' sentence frame and recount to adult
- Adopt appropriate position and posture for gaining adults' attention
- Enter conversation at appropriate point and recognise turns
- Copy accurately from model words and attempt to write simple regular words
- In books, use picture clues to guess a word and predict others
- Enjoy simple readers and picture books, and be able to talk about the story sequence

Adult strategies

- Control noise levels and distractions within listening environment
- Use physical prompts to gain child's attention before giving a message
- Provide contextually-based opportunities for language interaction so that there is little possibility of misunderstanding
- Liaise between family, speech therapist, and other helping adults so that activities can be consistently followed through
- When meaning miscarries give forced alternatives – 'Is it a blue duck or a blue swan?'
- Allow child time to respond without over-questioning or controlling conversation
- Avoid drawing attention to or correcting errors but provide a clear, distinct model in reply
- Paraphrase child's contribution and allow child to acknowledge the interpretation – 'It's too stiff, is it?'
- Provide opportunities for child to take the adult's role in pretend play, giving out materials
- In music and movement give rhythm exercises including dancing, walking, and skipping to a beat
- Encourage language courtesies, such as appropriate ways to gain adults' attention, correct posture and physical proximity when making requests or purchases, greeting, and thanking people
- Use joint story composition, using a word-processor or 'Breakthrough' materials, as a basis for shared discussion
- Accompany some messages with body gestures and non-verbal signals to reinforce meaning
- Read stories together, encourage sensible guesswork, commentary, and prediction

Teaching objectives for a secondary-aged child with specific language disorder

Description of child

>At 12 years of age Simon is confused by complex sentences. His own speech becomes unintelligible when he tries to produce a long sequence, and this is likely to have many confusions in syntax and word structure. He spends approximately 50 per cent of his time in mainstream classes with a range of adult supports, and the rest of the time in a language unit. In some practical areas such as rural science, cookery, and woodwork, he shows aptitude. He enjoys creating computer graphics, took part in a swimming display, and won an art

prize during the year. Socially competent, Simon gives the impression that he understands more than he does and this is highlighted when he has to read or write. Self-esteem is sometimes low.

Teaching objectives

- Take responsibility for being in the right place at the right time with correct books, and sitting in good listening position
- Ask for help when misunderstandings arise
- Be socially confident to ask for information, materials and services from adult using sentences
- Sustain attention for most of a lesson with some adult help
- Use concepts of time, weight, length, height, and comparatives such as more, same, equal, less
- Generate spoken and written language with help, to express opinions and feelings, ask questions and give information
- Be able to read a passage to locate a point of information or main idea, and summarise content
- Read a simple story and relate the sequence of ideas or events
- Use timetables, dictionary, catalogues, brochures, directories, maps, and encyclopaedias, to find information
- Join in informal activities in mainstream, such as sports clubs, interest groups, drama, and music
- Address adults and peers appropriately, e.g. enter conversation at proper point, use correct forms of address
- Use complex sentences in writing, including cohesive ties such as 'so', 'but', 'then', 'next'
- Use meaning-oriented reading strategies such as sensible prediction, cross-checking, and multi-cue sources
- Monitor own errors in reading and spelling, and have appropriate correction/inspection strategies
- Follow a sequence of detailed instructions, although written help or adult prompts may be needed

Adult strategies

- Create opportunities for small group or individual work every day using additional help/room management techniques
- Use topic work as a shared basis for language interaction since open-ended discussion may lead to breakdown in understanding
- Encourage use of language for describing experiences, asking questions, expressing feelings, passing on information, making judgements and predictions, categorising and analysing evidence
- Seize opportunities to reinforce child's successful language exchanges – 'Simon told me I forgot to lock the door.'

- Assess areas of curriculum where child may require pretutoring, help within the classroom and later reinforcement. Negotiate an appropriate timetable
- Co-ordinate the work of support staff, subject teachers, language specialists, and liaise with parents. Regular meetings should be held to monitor progress across the curriculum
- Give opportunity for exchange of roles in language work – 'I ask you/you ask me'
- Work on study skills such as locating information using contents, index, and headings, particularly where subject text-books are difficult
- Use computer software which provides a joint social context whereby adult and child interact around the program content
- Provide opportunities for the child to extend use of language outside the concrete here and now, in creative or imaginary work
- Choose books and materials which reflect the child's interests, experience and competence
- Provide written assignments or lesson plans to reinforce independent learning
- Do not assume comprehension and give opportunities for confirmation and cross-checking of understanding
- Avoid correcting faulty sentence structures, use paraphrase and restatement to provide a better model
- Create a consistent and positive atmosphere in which mistakes can be made without fear of ridicule or criticism
- Use opportunities which arise intrinsically from the child's experience across the curriculum to enrich the child's language awareness – 'Can you feel the water behind, or in front of your leg when you kick?'
- Raise expectations gradually, foster self-esteem by looking back at earlier work from time to time and recognising child's progress *with* the child

CURRICULUM PLANNING

For the child with language difficulties, early discussions should address the availability of adult supports and physical resources, such as the listening environment, together with a suitable programme of teaching objectives, stemming from a careful appraisal of the child's educational needs. The next step is to examine how the child's needs can be met within the curriculum of the school. In fact, curriculum planning may be the cornerstone of a successful integration programme for each child. The basic question for children with special needs revolves around which areas of the school curriculum the child has access to, is withdrawn from, or can participate in through adaptation. Who is going to be responsible for the 'core' curriculum of numeracy, literacy, science, and humanities? Is the curriculum wide enough, or will the child be spending almost all of the time on language and literacy work? Does the language specialist view the role as one of taking over specific areas of the curriculum, or of handing on strategies to the teachers in mainstream? If the former, there is a danger that the ordinary class teachers will view their own contributions as peripheral, not really important in the child's learning experience, other than in providing an opportunity for social contact with normal peers. If the latter, then time must be found to share ideas amongst class teachers and specialist support staff, at regular intervals. Once again this is a question of balance. The likely demands of each area of the curriculum will need to be looked at in turn. We should be careful, too, in assuming that a child will be able to participate without any modification or preparation in practical subjects such as art and craft, or in less formal areas such as movement and drama.

Decisions about curriculum, where and how a child is going to take part alongside peers, should be a shared endeavour taking into account the child's current achievements and learning skills, in relation to the challenges which are likely to be met in the mainstream class. Does the class teacher use formal teaching strategies with a heavy dependence on reading and recording skills, and can the teacher's approach be adapted easily? Will the child have to listen for long periods of time? Will there be a lot of new, unfamiliar or abstract terminology? Is the teacher going to use ways of presenting material, such as pie charts, graphs or bar diagrams, which may not have been met before? Which lessons have more practical, experiential content, and a less abstruse range of concepts? Children with speech and language difficulties may be much less confident in participating in a lesson involving a lot of oral discussion, the rote learning of facts, and work mainly done from textbooks, printed worksheets, or from blackboard presentations.

Some teachers are able to plan ahead in a degree of detail, if only in certain areas of the curriculum such as history, geography, and mathematics, where teaching may be topic-based. However, it is important to know what materials, information, concepts, and skills, the teacher is going to introduce over a period of time, and where any cross-curriculum links might be made. This kind of analysis can be used as a basis for devising a child's timetable and planning which subjects are to be taken in mainstream. Where it is felt that some areas of the school curriculum may be too demanding, the range of activities the child can join in with may need to be reduced in co-ordination with the extra help available.

Close, continuing contact between class teacher and supporting adults enables useful, day-to-day preparations to be made before a child joins in a mainstream class session. It may not always be necessary to pre-tutor every child in this way for every lesson. For the child with a language problem there is more likelihood of following and understanding a lesson, and of keeping pace with peers, if concepts have been introduced beforehand and a knowledge-base prepared. The content area can be gone over, any new or specialised vocabulary can be discussed, and links can be made with other areas of the child's schoolwork in advance. At the end of a lesson, support can be geared towards reinforcing the content covered, checking on what the child has actually taken in and understood, and filling in any gaps in comprehension or practising important skills further. To do all this successfully each of the adults involved with the child, including mainstream class teachers and supporting adults, needs to know what has been planned in an area of the curriculum and then covered. Some teachers keep a daily notebook which is passed backwards and forwards between class teacher and support staff. Parents can also be included in the circulation of this daily notebook, so that they too know what the child has been doing in class and can add their encouragement and help at home. Some schools feel a better policy is to select certain of the more interesting aspects of the child's school day for the parents to see and work over at home.

In all that has been said about curriculum planning an assumption is made that teachers will keep *relevance* to the fore. We live in a society of increasing leisure time and diminishing work opportunities. If a child's communication difficulties are to preclude some vocational and social outlets, it is all the more important that the child's school experience is a preparation for life after school. Of course this issue is paramount in the secondary stage. For children with speech and language problems, how we teach should aim to promote social confidence, acceptance and self-esteem. Appropriate attitudes to work, sex, and ethnic minorities are fostered in school. What we teach in the later years should lead up to work and leisure pursuits. 'Life' or 'survival' skills cut across subject boundaries but include some awareness of handling money, shopping and budgeting, using public transport, renting a flat, buying a house, hire purchase, insurance, wages and tax, paying gas and electricity bills, running a motorbike or car. It will also be particularly important for children with communication needs to be well-prepared in the subtleties of social relationships, love and marriage, family life and the responsibilities which accompany sexual experience.

THE HOME–SCHOOL BOOK

Parents often do not know how to use their energies most productively at home in sympathy with what the school staff are trying to achieve. A home–school notebook is especially helpful for young children with poor communication who find it hard to describe what they have been doing at school. The teacher highlights the main activities of the day, with suggestions for follow-up reading or discussion at home. Any newly discovered words or important ideas can be noted. Such a home–school diary also gives the parents an opportunity to mention special events at home, in anticipation of a visit to the hospital or dentist's, or a coming family milestone (a new baby or house move, for example), which generally enhances the links between family and school. In this way teachers can also relate classroom activities to significant experiences at home. One factor noted by Tizard and Hughes (1984), which was discussed in chapter 2, is that schools do not always supplement or reflect the child's experiences in the family. For some this results in alienation.

A home–school book is thus one way of bridging the gap between what the child does at home and in class. It can also function as a forward planner so that parents and teachers can prepare a child for new, exciting or potentially anxiety-raising experiences. Later on in this chapter we shall be examining other ways of sharing useful information between home and school, such as handing on effective strategies for communication.

THE PLAY CONTEXT

With young children at the nursery or early infant stage, the play context provides the most important informal opportunities for language use. There is a wealth of play materials and equipment designed for young children and most schools will have a wide choice of things which children will never have met before, and which they can discover and enjoy. However, it is not enough simply to set out an array of materials and then expect children to play productively. It is the contribution made by the adult towards creating the right atmosphere and opportunities for play, which is important. These issues have been looked into in a Schools Council Project (Manning and Sharp, 1977). Actually, the title of this book, *Structuring Play in the Early Years at School*, is misleading, because it suggests that adults must deliberately structure children's play activities. What is more usefully conveyed in the book, however, is that adults can shape play by careful selection of materials, subtle management of group situations, and by knowing when and how to join in.

What kind of play resources can be recommended for children with language difficulties? In chapter 2 we described some of Piaget's proposals on the development of thinking and its relation to language. In his view it is achievements in the early 'sensori-motor' period which make play possible. The child is first preoccupied with physical exploration – finding out what things feel like, how they work and what can be done with them. It follows that early sensori-motor play is usually concerned with investigating the qualities of everyday household objects, such as a pan, brush or spoon, by grasping, use of the mouth, and visual inspection. Out of this experience arises the awareness that objects exist outside the child and continue to do so, even when temporarily out of sight. Before long, the infant fits patterns of behaviour ('schemata') to appropriate objects. Cups and spoons may be put together and both used in self-feeding play. Towards the end of the sensori-motor period the child learns that one object can be used to represent another. The child may then brush a doll's hair or play at feeding a teddy with the cup and spoon. As symbolic awareness grows, the child is able to understand symbols of an increasingly arbitrary nature. Instead of life-size objects, the child is able to play appropriately with Wendy-House-sized materials, then objects suitable for a doll's house. Eventually, the child is able to play with toys which bear little perceptual similarity to the objects they represent, such as miniature cars. An understanding of two-dimensional symbols, such as pictures, is an indication that a child's symbolic development is well established. Verbal language, of course, is the stage of symbolic thinking where the word acts as a truly arbitrary symbol.

In the early stages it is important to provide toys and materials which foster symbolic play, at the level achieved by the child. Toys such as pegboards, shape puzzles, postboxes, formboards, containers, coloured beads, and blocks, are designed to establish fine manipulative skills and concepts of colour, shape and size. More helpful for imaginative play are versatile toys which can be used representationally. There are many kinds of construction materials available commercially, which can be fitted together to build vehicles, people, houses, farmyards, and space stations: some require more dexterity than others. Materials such as sand, drinking-straws, wood, eggboxes, coloured paper, plastic cartons, cardboard containers, plasticine, clay, and polystyrene can be used freely and adaptively in symbolic play. Other toys, such as garages, fire stations, forts, doll's houses, tea-sets, work-benches, train layouts, racetracks, zoos, military depots, hospitals, play schools and science fiction replicas, cultivate imaginary play, although in a more constrained and stereotyped way. As play develops, the properties of the materials themselves are less important in shaping the imaginary experience. Role play, or imitative play, reflects children's awareness of social roles as they act out recognisable characters and situations, such as parents and babies, doctors and nurses, cops and robbers, teacher and child, mums and dads, or cowboys and indians. Role play can be encouraged by small 'stage sets' with 'props', such as the Wendy-House, grocery counter, take-away food shop, or Post Office. Dressing-up clothes, especially hats, come in useful. Children can play-act familiar events, nursery rhymes, or stories, using finger- and glove-puppets, as well as dolls. Multi-media methods of representing a particular experience, such as a trip to a farmyard or bus depot, including model-making, role play, puppet acting, rhymes, songs, pictures, and of course talk, may help the child who requires repetition of new concepts and vocabulary, and who may have difficulty grasping a sequence of events.

The Schools Council Project on play, mentioned earlier (Manning and Sharp, 1977), suggests that adults sometimes direct, dominate and intervene too early in children's play. The issue of adult control is an important one to which we shall return in discussing conversation strategies. In the play context adults participate most effectively *alongside* children, perhaps suggesting new possibilities in the play experience, introducing different materials or information, without controlling the situation. In the same way that an adult may rephrase and expand a child's speech, so too, the adult can interpret and develop a child's play, working from the child's own ideas. The adult's management skills come into service in subtle ways: deciding which children make a viable group, and when a play situation is in danger of being disrupted. In a mainstream class the child with severe communication difficulties will need paired play to start with, in partnership with a non-threatening, peer-oriented agemate. If there is a danger of materials being misused, of a conflict of interests, or of one child disturbing the play of a small group, more positive direction and control may be called for from the adult. As a source book the work of Manning and Sharp (1977) has some helpful suggestions about domestic play, natural materials, outdoor play, play-acting and constructional play. Adults are asked to think about the purpose and intention of play for the child, how further possibilities can be drawn out, and when adults need to be more directly involved. The books by Garvey (1977) and Jeffree, McConkey, and Hewson (1977) also present a range of practical pointers. A distinctive feature, which most of these recent studies highlight, is the co-ordination of activity which children achieve in the play task. Even children with very limited language resources, whose play is constrained to the concrete 'here and now', will usually be stimulated by the social momentum of a shared play context to assert their intentions and plan their thinking.

TURN-TAKING

There is one particular social convention which is fundamental to effective communication, and that is knowing when to speak and when to listen. The framework within which conversation takes place has some very early prototypes in the turn-taking patterns of mother–baby interactions. Bruner (1975) and Schaffer (1977) suggest that alternate exchanges, when first the parent and then the baby responds, are important for later reciprocal interactions in dialogue. There are several play routines, too, which give children the experience of turn-taking. These play episodes may be useful for young children with language difficulties to rehearse in school. Back-and-forth games with beanbags, marbles, cars, and battery driven vehicles are enjoyable. Children are equally enthusiastic about taking turns to post shapes, shake dice, pick cards, and make moves in board games; as well as more boisterous turn-taking in relays, musical stops, and 'Simple Simon' action routines. Nursery rhymes also provide opportunities for children to listen and join in at the correct moment, such as 'Ring a ring of roses' and 'London Bridge is falling down'.

For older children, role play or direct experience can be arranged so that children can practise appropriate posture and physical proximity when addressing others; greeting adults, unfamiliar and familiar; starting and finishing talking; asking questions; making requests and giving thanks; making an order or purchase; asking for help; passing on messages; and speaking clearly to groups. Particularly important for many children is knowing how to gain an adult's attention, when a need is pressing. Using 'walkie-talkies' and telephones also gives useful experience of conversational exchange, even if that is limited to 'Hello' and 'Goodbye'.

ATTENTION AND LISTENING

The ability to attend to a stimulus, to ignore distractions, and to listen over a period of time involves a complex hierarchy of skills. Sensory information has to be taken in selectively, organised, and then interpreted. At a very basic level children have to select the important sound contrasts from the stream of speech used around them. From the early stages onwards children share a frame of reference in which visual attention to people and objects, the social meaning of a situation, and linguistic stimuli, are integrated. Attention can be disrupted in a number of ways: at the sensory input level, through auditory or visual impairments; at the cognitive level, because of failure to categorise, or make sense of information; at the psychological level, related to motivation, emotional arousal and competing interests; finally, there may be medical factors, such as medication or tiredness, which interfere with concentration. Poor attention control will greatly hamper a child's development of language. Having acquired language, words themselves serve to direct attention and mediate experience.

There is one approach to language intervention which starts off from the basis that language-handicapped children manifest attention problems (Cooper, Moodley, and Reynell, 1978). These authors describe a number of clear stages in the normal development of attention control, with activities to promote skills at each level. To begin with, all infants are extremely distractible, paying only fleeting attention to every new stimulus. For children at this stage the learning task must be the dominant stimulus and distractions kept to a minimum. Later on, children can concentrate for longer, but cannot tolerate interruptions. Tasks have to be self-evident, since verbal instructions or rewards intrude. At the next stage, attention is more flexible, but a child would not yet be able to listen to an adult's directions whilst concentrating on a toy. Before delivering an instruction, it is necessary to stop the child's current activity. Later still, children become capable of controlling their own attention focus, switching from listening to looking, but not both simultaneously. Children still have to focus their full concentration on a verbal or visual source. In the final stages, multi-channel attention is established. At this mature point instructions can be delivered whilst the child is engaged in something else: an experiment can be watched to a spoken accompaniment, whilst the child is expected to take notes.

This stage analysis of attention control has important implications for the teaching context. We have already mentioned the value of sympathetic acoustic conditions. For children in the early stages, tasks should be kept short, material and activities should be presented separately, and with as few distractions as possible. Before initiating conversation, attention can be caught by a touch on the elbow, calling the child's name or establishing eye contact. It should be remembered that children may need help to shift from one activity to another and that clear directions must be given before, not during, an activity when the child's whole attention is on the adult. There are several group games which foster listening, starting with simple location and identification tasks. Children can be asked to indicate, with eyes shut, where selected sounds are coming from, such as a clock, tambourine or drum. A variation of hide-and-seek can be played where the adult makes sounds softer or louder as the child approaches or goes further away from a hidden object. In identification games children are asked to identify sounds of different objects or instruments. Sound effects, such as running water, ambulance, doorbell, telephone, washing machine, motorbike, vacuum cleaner or bacon frying, can be presented on tape.

The most significant development in achieving mature attention is the transfer of focus from one stimulus to another which gradually comes under the child's control. As this is achieved individuals are able to work alongside others in small groups and can tolerate more interruptions and distractions. Adults may wish to decrease the number of physical prompts to gain the child's attention and use verbal prompts instead, such as the child's name or 'Watch me', 'Listen', 'Stop what you're doing and look up.' Similarly, the child may increasingly be expected to cope with an instruction or question whilst absorbed in something else. Listening games for children at these stages can be more complex. For example, children can be asked to select a particular object or toy from an array, and then follow a simple instruction: 'Make the brown horse run.' In 'Eligibility' children are asked to perform an action, such as nodding their heads, if they have red shoes, blue jumpers, long hair, and so on. Children can be asked to listen out for their names, silly mistakes, objects or particular words, in stories. One very helpful set of activities for children who have a poor rhythmical foundation for language is to present familiar rhymes and jingles with pauses for children to fill in missing words. A rhythm or sequence of sounds, beats and claps can be given for the child to model. 'Musical stops' requires children to listen for a particular rhythm, drum beat or stop in the music, at which point everybody sits down, makes statues or plays dead.

Finally, adult support to attention-focus can be faded as attention is integrated across sensory channels and sustained for longer periods. At this stage children can work in large groups, listen to instructions with a greater information load whilst engaged in another activity, and follow a sequence of set tasks. Concentration and listening may be extended through auditory awareness and recall tasks. One popular activity starts with an adult giving a sequence of directions for drawings which increase in complexity. For example: 'Draw a house with a tree to the right'; then: 'Put a red car next to a blue sign with green capital letters on it', and so on.

Gossip games involve passing messages from child to child, or relating and then enlarging story sequences or sets of instructions. There are many ideas for practising sound awareness. For example, a taped or spoken sound can be presented, followed by a word containing the sound. Children are asked whether the sound occurs at the beginning, middle, or end of the word. Sound games include: 'I spy'; putting orally given words into sound families, such as bread, said, red; detecting rhymes or alliteration; making sound blends and spoonerisms. In chapter 3 we mentioned the conviction amongst some dyslexia theorists that children who are good at recognising sounds and have an ear for rhythms, rhymes and alliterations make better readers. Listening skills are part of a spectrum of language-related behaviours which underpin literacy. Further suggestions for listening games can be found in Jeffree and McConkey (1976), or Webster and Ellwood (1985).

CONVERSATION STRATEGIES

Perhaps the most important way in which children with speech and language difficulties may be helped is through an awareness of how adults can stimulate and facilitate language interaction. There is a growing body of evidence, which was reviewed in chapter 2, that children are active in their discovery of language and use their experience of interaction with other speakers to construct and test out their own representations of the language system. Conversation in shared contexts of purposeful and meaningful activity, provides a well-tailored source of evidence from which children can learn. Of course, some children give fewer cues to adults and are less good at initiating interaction. On the other hand, adults also vary in their responsiveness. There is a range of modifications which adults can make to their own styles of responding which both enhance and sustain language interaction. Interactional experiences which are rich and facilitative would appear to be crucial for children with difficulties in learning to communicate.

What intentions do adults realise in adjusting their speech to children? In the first place, adults try (without being fully aware of it) to improve the child's access to the language system. Almost all of the features of adults' speech to infants, summarised in chapter 2, serve to gain the child's attention, simplify the patterns of language used, and clarify what is said through devices such as repetition and clear pronunciation. A second set of strategies is geared towards mutual comprehension, such as expanding and paraphrasing what the child says. The third kind of modifications which adults make sustains the child's participation in conversation, for example, by relating what is said to previous utterances and inviting the child to say more. It is the second and third types of strategy which appear to be most helpful in accelerating children's language learning (Wells, 1985), and these will be considered in some detail. A summary of the strategies felt to be either more or less helpful in language interactions with children in school is given in table 5.2.

Mutual comprehension is most easily secured when commentary surrounds a joint activity, the child's immediate play, or a shared imaginary experience, such as a story. The adult's responses reflect and develop the topic of interest, perhaps by adding further information, or drawing attention to other aspects of the situation which might be relevant. The child is allowed to initiate a high proportion of interactions, whilst the adult follows the child's lead, rather than directing the activity. The child is encouraged to question and search out possibilities. A less effective style is where the adult tends to initiate new topics and to pursue them at the expense of themes the child might wish to introduce. Responsive adults monitor the child's responses carefully, restating and expanding what the child says. Input is provided which is finely tuned to the child's interests and behaviour. Sentences are tailored to the child's level of understanding, providing a more explicit and elaborate version, not too far apart structurally from the child's, and incorporating elements of the previous contribution:

Child: Kitty scratch.
Adult: Yes, Kitty scratched your arm.
Child: We undoned it.
Adult: We undid your button ... to see your scratch.

Thus, the child's intended meaning is interpreted and checked. An opportunity is given to confirm or reject the interpretation which is negotiated between the participants, in relation to the language context. The adult's rewording provides a better syntax model, without any sense of correction, and without losing sight of the function of the child's language use. Further examples of this kind of adult responsiveness, in both home and school contexts, have been given in chapter 2.

Strategies which sustain the child's involvement include showing a genuine interest in what the child has to say, handing conversation back to the child after every turn, and allowing time for a reply. The adult avoids dominating, controlling, correcting, or finishing off what the child is trying to say. Responses such as 'Well I never', 'Oh yes', 'sounds great', provide conversational oil and invite the child to add more. So too, when adults give

Table 5.2 *Conversation strategies in the classroom*

Helpful	Less helpful
Giving commentary on the child's play and activity, showing an interest in what the child is doing, helping the child to understand more about the chosen topic.	Over use of 'open' questions such as 'What did you do at the weekend?' (closed questions are more likely to receive a response, even if only Yes/No).
Allowing the child to question, giving information and explanation.	Asking for information which the adult already possesses – 'What colour is your T-shirt?' (test questions).
Expanding, paraphrasing, and clarifying the child's intended meaning.	Enforcing the child to repeat a correct model – 'Say "I went", not "I goed".'
Listening to what the child has to say, allowing the child to introduce new topics, giving eye contact and signalling attention.	Asking the child to imitate a correct sentence or correcting faulty pronunciation ('frog, not shog').
Handing conversation back to the child each time and waiting for the child to reply. Avoiding dominating the interchange.	Talking *for* the child – not giving time for the child to respond.
Sharing experiences, both practical and imaginative, as a basis for talking *with* the child.	Trying deliberately to teach language, vocabulary or correct grammar out of context. ('Today, we are going to learn the names of things you find in a bathroom.')
Providing social oil to sustain interaction – 'Hm, that's interesting.'	Managing, dominating, or controlling comments are less helpful to young children in sustaining dialogue.
Giving personal contributions – 'Yesterday, I went to …'	Responses which discourage the child's exploration and confidence – approval and interest in appropriate activities are the key.

something to the dialogue from their own personal experience, the child is stimulated to contribute further.

Questions have to be considered carefully. We know from the Tizard and Hughes (1984) work that questioning is an important aspect of language interaction, more so when it is the *child* who initiates the enquiry. In joint activities with adults, children are often observed asking how items work, where people are going and what things mean. With many children, everything that is said demands a response of some kind from an adult. However, some adult moves lead to a decrease in spontaneous language from children, and overquestioning *by the adult* is an example. Open questions, such as 'What did you do at school today?', 'What happened next?', 'What can you see in the picture?', are intended simply to elicit speech and often fail. Open questions offer no help to the child in formulating a reply. In the same vein, children usually sense when they are being tested out by display questions, to which the adult already knows the answers. If the adult must interrogate, closed questions relating to a current activity will provide easier slots for a child to fill in reply, even if this is restricted to 'Yes' or 'No'.

DIRECT TEACHING TECHNIQUES

There is a view that children who experience language learning difficulties can be trained on specific points of language. In chapter 4 we looked at some of the commercial materials which claim to identify gaps in a child's language skills and set about to remediate them through exercises and drills. Of necessity, the focus of direct teaching and rehearsal techniques shifts away from the social context of language interaction towards the *form* of language. Less emphasis is placed on the function and meaning of language, rooted in shared experience, whilst more attention is paid to the structure of language *per se*, such as word endings or syntax patterns.

A number of research studies have shown that children with special needs have a double disadvantage in that they may be less well disposed to enter language interactions or to elicit responsive behaviour from adults. Less nurturing language encounters may exacerbate a child's primary learning difficulties. Wood, Wood, Griffiths and Howarth (1986) have found that adults' difficulties in communicating with deaf children lead them to adopt highly controlling and didactic strategies. They try to elicit language forms, teach new vocabulary, and spend a lot of time prompting children to imitate exemplary phrases, whilst correcting errors. Similar findings have been reported for children with other handicapping conditions, such as Down's syndrome. Mitchell (1976) reports a greater tendency for adults to command, control and prohibit Down's children, to ask more display questions and give more physical prompts. It is argued that these strategies are equally counterproductive for children with or without special needs.

Bearing these reservations in mind, let us turn to some of the techniques which are sometimes used to rehearse selected aspects of language. Imitation procedures require the child to repeat an adult sentence model, following an instruction such as 'Say after me...' A series of imitation tasks, with a gradual increase in sentence complexity, could be given to the child in this way. However, we know that children learn most effectively by discovering for themselves the underlying principles of language. In imitation tasks we cannot be sure a language rule has been acquired and then used to reconstruct an utterance, since the child may just be mimicking, parrot-fashion. The classic example, which shows that children can only imitate *within* the constraints of their existing language competence, was given by McNeill (1966, page 69):

Child: Nobody don't like me.
Mother: No, say 'Nobody likes me.'
Child: Nobody don't like me.
(8 repetitions of this dialogue)
Mother: No, listen carefully, say 'Nobody likes me.'
Child: Oh, nobody don't likes me.

Another common imitation strategy is used to elicit a response, usually with picture stimuli or in a game context, whereby the adult provides most of the sentence pattern. For example, the adult might pick up a card and say 'I've got a bicycle', and each child uses the same structure with a change in vocabulary, as turns are taken. Other drills include forced alternatives where the child has to make a choice and generate a new sentence, although most of the sentence pattern is given: 'Is Jane *kissing* the teddy or *hitting* the teddy?'; 'Is it *in* the box, or *on* the box?' In cloze strategies the child is given a sentence framework with just the gaps to consider, whilst a prompt is given through a rise in intonation: 'There's a big, red...; it lives in a...'

A body of techniques has been devised to teach specific aspects of receptive and expressive language. An extensive summary is given in the practical guidelines devised by Cooke and Williams (1985). In a typical set-piece, these authors describe how prepositions can be taught. The child is given a toy bed, a toy table and a small doll, with the instruction 'Put the doll *under* the *table*.' The key words are stressed, and the adult provides feedback and repetition. Gradually the number of possible locations are increased (bed, chair, bath), whilst the number of subject choices is extended (man, girl, baby). The complexity of attribute terms can also be increased (small blue doll, big red table). In another set-piece, verbs are taught by making teddies and dolls carry out actions in response to verbal instructions such as dance, walk, run, and wave. Commands, using puppets, objects, and locations, are made increasingly complex. Alternatively, aspects of language can be illustrated using pictures; storyboards with movable pictures; action people; floor layouts of scenes such as a street, park or hospital; and other miniature toy scenarios.

Several points should be borne in mind when language is taught, however ingenious the methods may seem. Firstly, in most spontaneous communication settings it is the *child*, not the adult, who takes the initiative. It is the child who is active and who shares control in searching out the meaning of a context through language. This paradigm is reversed when the adult is didactic and controlling, seeking to develop meanings or hand over information which has importance for the teacher. Secondly, language has an impetus which stems from real purpose inherent in the activity. There must be a genuine pressure to communicate, hard to sustain in contrived contexts. In a speech-clinic setting, the child must often be aware that the underlying purpose of the exercise is that the adult wants the child to use new and different language forms. Thirdly, in natural language contexts anything which disrupts the flow of conversation is constraining, such as excessive use of questions, commands or corrections. There is a real danger, then, that the child with difficulties in speech and language will interpret most direct elicitation techniques, drills and set-pieces, quite correctly, as prompts to talk.

LANGUAGE ACROSS THE CURRICULUM

As Halliday (1975) has pointed out, language is both system *and* resource. In other words, children learn language through using it, and in school, language is a means to learn other things. In this section we set out to explore how language enrichment opportunities arise *intrinsically* from the curriculum. The term 'language across the curriculum' was popularised by the Bullock Report (DES, 1975) and some would say that, of all the recommendations made in this report, the concepts behind such a language policy are the most far reaching. There are many ways in which ideas specifically recommended for children with special needs also reflect good practice for all children. Helping children to use language more productively in school is a case in point. At the heart of the Bullock argument is the view that all genuine learning engages the child in a process of discovery. Knowledge is never simply passed on from adult to child: 'What is known must in fact be brought to life afresh within every 'knower' by his own efforts.' (Op. cit., page 50.) For children with speech and language difficulties it is important to seize all the opportunities presented in school, across the subject boundaries, where children are involved in talking, listening, questioning, reading and writing, as a means to help children actively uncover more about language itself.

What role does the teacher have? In keeping with all that has been said in this book about conditions for learning, the role is less to do with handing over something that the teacher has, and much more to do with shaping experiences in which children reconstruct knowledge for themselves, and build onto what they already understand. Prompting children to use language in order to extend their own learning is not simply a matter of deploying a set of techniques, for example, in sustaining conversation. It is also a matter of being aware of ways of working which foster reflective, independent enquiry. There is, for example, a stark contrast between teaching from set texts, comprehension cards or work-sheets, and an approach which encourages children to collect their own observations, organise findings, explain their own confusions, and weigh evidence in order to reach solutions. Good teaching practice is based on an awareness of the multiplicity of purposes, described in chapter 1, to which language can be put.

Teaching often begins by the marking out of a relevant area of interest. The greatest impact is usually achieved by presenting topics through real-life experiences. A teacher in a language unit known to the authors prefaces all her important topics with an *actual* visit, for example, to a churchyard, fire-station, farm, shop, factory, airport, brewery, Roman fort, railway station, building site, stables, canal lock, market, pond, depending on what is nearby. Where the teacher wants to use more remote subject matter, these are brought to life as far as possible by using artefacts, materials or pictures. Working with nursery and infant children, Dowling (1980) describes a number of projects where the teacher introduces a topic carefully and guides the children's exploration in order to enrich their thinking and language. The starting point for a project on people is a photograph of the teacher as a baby and the group is asked to bring in similar pictures of themselves. A mother is invited to feed or bath the baby with the children watching. This stimulates the class into activities related to size, food, and growth. Some children collect baby items to emphasise their relative smallness.

Others find pictures to illustrate an infant's development over time. Using a mirror the children are asked to observe similarities and differences in their own body sizes, hair, skin, and eyes. This leads on to an investigation of how faces register feelings, and contrasts such as young/old, lively/sleepy, angry/peaceful, love/hurt, or bored/interested.

The teacher is not just providing a stimulus, because what follows must have purpose and relevance. Blank (1985) argues that if topics are presented to children in terms of categories, such as weather, sounds, colours, shapes, quantities, texture, vehicles, holidays, and the like, then children will tend to be constrained in their thinking and language to the merely descriptive. A more effective approach in fostering dialogue, exploration, and exchange of ideas, is to introduce what Blank calls the 'predicated concept' (op. cit., page 16). Put simply, that means topics are introduced by a noun plus a predicate. In place of babies, we might put 'feeding babies' which is more likely to lead children to hypothesise about babies' dependency on adults, why infants require warm milk and how they are weaned. Young children are inevitably interested in their own bodies, their families and the immediate environment. 'Predicated topics', such as moving house, going to school, buying food, making the dinner, going to work, shape the way in which children organise their observations and analysis, and record data. The teacher introduces additional material and activities, such as stories, poems, tapes, TV program-mes, visits, movement, and role-play, as and when appropriate, in order to sharpen or widen the focus.

The book by Dowling (1980) is a very useful source of ideas for young children, covering topics such as where people and animals live; different occupations such as delivering the post, driving buses, cleaning windows, the police force, doctors and nurses; how and why people travel; what people wear and the reasons for different kinds of clothing; together with a host of suggestions relating to the natural environment: looking after animals, growing things, watching birds. The golden rule is to start with the familiar and move outwards. In what she describes as an 'object lesson', Rosen (1971) gives an entertaining account of how she taught 'the Normans' as an interesting story from the past, but one which her children were unable to relate to themselves or their lives. As a rethink, Rosen then took her class to an old windmill, where the children took rubbings of the surfaces of the mill-stones, examined the sail-fixings and took photographs of the buildings. The experience heralded investigations into mill-construction; different kinds of millstones, flour and bread; whilst a 'Miller' in the group prompted a discussion of surnames.

Another important principle is that it may not always be the formal teaching contexts which give rise to the most productive language interaction. In the book by Tizard and Hughes (1984) it is apparent that when adults converse with their children at home, the context is often banal. Some of the richest exchanges arose out of mundane chores such as washing-up and sorting out clothes. However, adults in school may feel that these are *not* valuable opportunities for talk: one activity may be cleared away efficiently by a lone adult, in order to move quickly onto the next set task. It could be argued that question forms emerge genuinely in contexts where children are sharing out materials and equipment and have to ask for what they need. In changing for games lessons, children have a natural demand for pronouns and possessives, in response to questions such as 'whose peg/coat/socks/shoes are these?' Putting toys, tools, books, and apparatus away, requires prepositions such as 'in', 'on', 'under', 'next to', 'below', 'in front of' and 'between'. Almost all children have an opportunity to enjoy cooking in school and the informal opportunities for discussion which this activity gives rise to are exemplary. A vocabulary for ingredients is required; together with action words, such as 'mix', 'melt', 'shake', 'stir', 'beat', 'sieve'; as well as a range of attribute terms to describe shape, taste, texture, or colour. Children use language in this kind of situation to direct, make requests, express reactions, and make their feelings known.

In a recent book, Hutt (1986) describes a number of aspects of the school curriculum, such as art and music, which are important parts of an overall approach to children with speech and language problems. Drawing, painting, and making, are obviously essential activities in fostering representational ability in children. Using materials of different colours and textures is not only an alternative means of self-expression, it is also a rich source of descriptive vocabulary, perceptual training and fine motor co-ordination practice. Children can depict emotions, are helped in their organisational skills, and can achieve confidence and relaxation in creative work. Similarly, drama can be used to help children listen attentively to instructions; take turns; show a variety of personal feelings through facial expressions, gestures, and tone of voice; and adopt roles in mime activities to develop 'pretend' sequences.

One of the observations often made about children with severe language difficulties is that general clumsiness, poor motor co-ordination and a limited rhythmical sense, are typical. A programme of physical education and movement, including skipping, jumping, catching balls, and using apparatus, may help children organise their movements, develop body perception, and rhythmical awareness as well as providing opportunities for using the language of body parts, space, position, and action. Music too, can provide experiences which foster auditory discrimination, memory, rhythm, and self-expression. Hutt (1986) describes a number of musical activities through which children are introduced to concepts such as long/short, quick/slow, loud/soft, high/low, angry/ peaceful, together with the subtler language of harmony and melody. Rhythmical exercises include repeating a drum rhythm, clapping the regular accent at the beginning of each bar, and walking and skipping in time. A melody played on an instrument can provide the rhythmical foundation for children to learn simple phrases and songs.

Mathematics and science are essential curriculum areas for children with communication difficulties. In many cases the concepts of these subject areas are within reach of the child, but the language of instruction is overwhelming. In the early stages of mathematics, concepts need to be related to everyday, concrete experience and particular care is required to use the language of quantity, capacity, area, length, weight and time, in meaningful contexts. In science the child's ability to set up hypotheses, make observations, categorise information and draw conclusions, both arise from and foster understanding of the language of enquiry. The skills involved in making comparisons (more, same, longer, biggest); in ordering (next, tomorrow, first, before); and in classifying (all, dead, dry, black) require precise vocabulary to shape precise thinking. Examples given by Robertson (1980) show how science enquiries depend for their success on the teacher helping children to develop effective strategies and information skills, from the initial ordering of their fact-finding, to the giving of a clear report for others to read. In one of her case studies, secondary-age children visited a graveyard which inspired youngsters to record the proportion of infant deaths in different historical periods. The teacher played an important part in helping children to work over their experience, set themselves questions, find supportive information and present their insights to others. The books by Robertson (1980) and Wray (1985) are very useful accounts of children at all levels, using curriculum-encounters to enrich their use of language. Ultimately, and this is a point emphasised by Donaldson (1978) and which was discussed in chapter 2 of this book, the child has to proceed to an abstract awareness of the learning process. Children require a sense of how to go about their learning; a capacity to think about their enquiry strategies; in other words, they need to learn how to learn.

READING, WRITING AND LANGUAGE

In this section, for the sake of simplicity, we have isolated aspects of literacy from children's wider use of language in the curriculum. That should not be taken to imply that we feel literacy should be taught as a subject set apart from the child's general learning experience. A well thought out curriculum must create the impulse for children to communicate through different modalities: speech, reading, and writing. Despite some obvious differences between the spoken and written forms of language, we shall be arguing that what children learn in their initial encounters with spoken language, is later applied to literacy. Furthermore, children approach the printed word with the same attitudes, learning styles, strategies, and purpose, which characterise their experience of oral communication. The same principles for teaching and interaction can be applied to spoken dialogue and written text. When adults set about helping children to read, much of what we have said about learning as a collaborative, meaning-oriented partnership, across the school curriculum, applies equally well to reading.

In the normal course of events children arrive in school as sophisticated spoken language users with a wealth of communication experience. Learning to read and write can be considered, at one level, as processes whereby the child acquires the printed code which represents speech. Normally, we would not expect children to grasp the complexities of the written word before their spoken abilities are well advanced. For children who experience communication difficulties the processes of learning to read and write present a dual problem. The child does not know the printed code. Nor are the aspects of language which the code represents well controlled. So the acquisition of literacy becomes a language-learning process at one and the same time. To some degree this is true of all children learning to read.

At another level, print extends the use of language into the 'disembedded mode', where there is no immediate context, apart from that established by the text itself, or through picture clues. The reader enters a different kind of partnership with the author from that normally experienced in a language dialogue. Features such as pitch, intonation, rhythm, and stress are often poorly registered in print. The help that the author has rooted in the text itself depends on the reader's prior language experience to recover. The negotiation of meaning, characterised in adult's talk to children by a range of finely-tuned adjustments and modifications, in writing can only take an imprecise account of the needs of the language novice, since the child is not present when the text is constructed. The importance of the written word is the limitless opportunity it gives for children to have access to information, to think creatively about concepts and ideas, to organise and challenge their understanding of the world beyond the 'here and now'. Written forms of language are inherently able to handle more complex and abstract data, than is speech. Evidence presented in a visual form can be scrutinised, dissected, and developed in a way which would overrun the fleeting presence of speech. In the school years increasing demands are made upon children, through books and written work, to treat language itself as a space in which problems can be set up, experimented with, evaluated, and resolved. The written word is the medium through which information, technology, and our cultural heritage is transmitted. It is also a means by which linguistic skills are practised and extended.

Researchers do not always agree on what children need to know about language, in the early stages, in order to read. In chapter 2 a model of the separate levels of the structure of language was presented, including the organisation of sounds, syntax, and meaning. Which of these aspects of language structure need to be well controlled before the child can embark on reading? Which aspects are of such central importance to reading that if they are only weakly established or immature, then reading may break down? Perhaps the most important question concerns the extent to which reading requires an *explicit* awareness of particular features of the language system. In other words, children must not only be able to use language in their day-to-day communication, they are also required to reflect on how the code itself is put together and how it works. Besides being language users, to what extent must children be aware of how the linguistic system operates? If we can provide answers to some of these questions we may then be able to understand the relationships between speech and language development on the one hand, and literacy on the other. Similarly, for children who experience problems in certain aspects of their language development, the part played by reading and writing in resolving them may also become clear.

'BOTTOM-UP' PROCESSES – DECODING TEXT

It has been fashionable in the last decade for reading theorists to talk about 'bottom-up' processes, 'top-down' processes, or a mixture of the two. The term 'bottom-up' suggests that reading begins at the level of the print on the page. The reader is sensitive to basic building blocks, such as letter shapes or word patterns, which are then pieced together. Reading is a process of working upwards from clues in the text until the meaning of the whole is eventually recovered. 'Top-down' processes stress what the reader brings to the task, rather than what is found there. The reader draws on a knowledge of language and the world in order to make hypotheses about what might be found in a text. Put another way, the reader looks for meaning, rather than letters or words. These reading routes are not mutually exclusive, and it could be argued that children may use both sources of information to find out what text means.

Let us now return to the language model in figure 2.1 (page 36). The left-hand side of this diagram identifies pronunciation features and how these may be set down in print. In terms of reading, the salient aspects are the 40 or so distinctive sound contrasts, known as phonemes, and the 26 alphabet letters which are used to write them down. Since there are not enough letters to match each sound contrast, the correspondence between phonemes and graphemes is not equivalent. Some words have a distinctive visual appearance, such as 'yacht' or 'eye', where the corresponding letter sounds hinder pronunciation. In other cases visually similar words, such as 'rough', 'bough' and 'though', sound very different. Despite the unpredictability of the English system, heavy emphasis has been placed on phoneme–grapheme decoding, in teaching children to read. It is argued that children need to be aware how speech can be split into separate speech segments. In the early stages of teaching, the child's attention is drawn to the regular, commonly occurring sound features, such as the individual consonants and vowels in words like 'web', 'dog', 'van'. Later, teaching may move onto sound blends in words like 'boil', 'dust', and 'pram', before finally identifying more complex clusters in words such as 'flight', 'throat', or 'gloom'. The argument runs that children who use such 'phonic' strategies are helped to discover the meaning of new words by pronouncing them aloud. There is said to be sufficient regularity in spelling patterns for children to learn by recognising similar sound sequences in words such as 'thread' and 'bread', or 'flick' and 'trick'.

Decoding to sound (or 'phonic') strategies are 'bottom-up' in the sense that children are encouraged to derive cues from the text in order to identify words. Reading instruction typically involves the rehearsal and drilling of phonic ground-rules, as separate activities from the business of reading proper. The child might be expected to have mastered a set of subskills, for example, in recognising letter shapes and sound sequences, before tackling books. Defenders of the phonic approach usually argue that good readers seem much more aware of these rules than do poor readers (Snowling, 1980). Having an ear for sounds, alliteration and rhymes seems to characterise children who read either very early, or very well (Clark, 1976). The reading difficulties experienced by hearing-impaired children have sometimes been ascribed to the problem of 'hearing sounds in words' (Conrad, 1979); whilst dyslexia theorists have also pin-pointed sound segmentation processes as a fundamental learning obstacle (Snowling, 1985).

When different remedial strategies for poor readers are compared, phonic programmes are usually claimed to be the most effective (Gittelman and Feingold, 1983). A critique of all this literature, within a developmental language model, has been given by Webster (1986a).

Teachers need to be aware of several points in considering how children's language skills become integrated with reading. Firstly, the pronunciation aspects of the language model in figure 2.1 occupy a peripheral position, less central in terms of the child's development, than control of syntax. Of course, the sound features of language and print provide important cues, but perhaps more important in understanding written language is good control of the organising principles of syntax. Secondly, there are many routes to reading, and 'bottom-up' strategies are but one example. For children with speech and language difficulties, the questions which need to be asked are how far a phonic route might be helpful or confusing, and how such a 'bottom-up' approach fits in with current views on language-learning in the wider sense. It goes without saying that many children, and for the variety of reasons outlined in chapter 3, may have difficulties at the sound level. For children with auditory discrimination problems, who find it difficult to disting-uish, categorise, and respond to sounds, then a phonic approach starts from the child's weakness. Children who are unable to discern the rhythmical basis of speech are unlikely to gain much from sound segmentation drills. Furthermore, any approach which rehearses subskills of reading in rote fashion, and in isolation from purposeful meaning-oriented reading tasks, runs counter to much of what we have said about language development in general. Reading for meaning, with the child as an active participant in the process, harnessing the child's natural strengths of enquiry, we shall consider later.

READING, GRAMMAR AND EXPECTANCY

It is the child's control of syntax which is central in determining whether a sentence pattern is understood, in both speech and print. In the course of normal development, children acquire the rules of syntax through conversational interaction with adults. In the 'to and fro' of social dialogue, adults provide just sufficient challenges in well-tailored responses to what the child says, which supplies evidence from which children actively construct their own gramma-tical rules. How far can reading enrich this process?

Some researchers have suggested that when children have severe difficulties in acquiring spoken language, written words can be used to introduce and reinforce simple vocabulary and grammar. In a project with deaf children, Söderbergh (1985) describes an approach where written words, together with signs or speech, are tied directly to the child's everyday experience around the home, eating, dressing, or going to school. A child having difficulty with words like 'slowly' or 'quickly', would play a running and walking game as illustration, whilst the printed words and spoken vocabulary are presented. Using this method the child is said to crack the written code and enrich spoken language at the same time. It is a moot point how far language can be introduced to children in this way. There are many children whose reading abilities fall behind oral language skills. There are few instances where the reverse occurs. The weight of opinion suggests that reading progress usually depends on prior, or parallel, developments in the child's spoken language experience. Children need to discover what language is, and what it does, in oral contexts, before learning to read.

Linguists sometimes refer to the principle of language 'expectancy' in the classroom. When stories are read and children are introduced to their first reading books, the language used should be compatible with the child's expectations. Where there is a large gap between the child's understanding of syntax and the grammatical complexity of reading materials, there may be serious comprehension problems. In the early stages, in order to benefit from the predictable nature of familiar language, children need to meet up with vocabulary and sentence patterns that they use in their spoken language. In fact, many reading schemes do not meet criteria for language expectancy, because they are based on the repetition of key vocabulary, or designed to highlight phonic rules. Sentence structures of the kind: 'See Dick, jump Dick, jump up high', or 'Pat the fat rat', foster the idea that reading is an alien verbal activity, unrelated to everyday language experience.

One approach which guarantees that reading materials reflect the interests and expectations of the child as a language user is for children to write their own first books. The starting point might be a story or picture stimulus, or perhaps an exciting experience. Children are then encouraged to relate their own stories, which may be taped and written down. 'Breakthrough' materials (Mackay, Thompson, and Schaub, 1970) are based on similar ideas. Children are given a vocabulary bank: a store of printed words relating to the child's interests, function words such as 'to', and action words such as 'go'. A special frame holds the cards on which the words are printed and this is used to compose sentences, which are later written down. For young children with speech and language difficulties, it is good practice to use reading materials which reflect the child's language experience, using vocabulary that is familiar, with sentence patterns not too far apart structurally, from those that the child has mastered. Some adults adapt appealing children's books by covering over complex text with a more linguistically appropriate 'gloss' or annotation, leaving the story structure and illustrations intact.

There may come a time, particularly with older children, when it is less helpful to restrict or modify the reading materials to which they are exposed. We have argued that there is no single route to reading, and children can be helped to search for alternative cue sources in text, beyond the syntax. In the section on independent reading we shall be looking at how children's attention can be drawn to the variety of information sources in books, such as dramatic structure, picture clues, likely events and storytime, together with cues rooted in the text. There is a danger in the deliberate simplification of reading materials that some of these potential cue sources are lost.

There are several ways in which the grammatical patterns of written sentences can be highlighted in order to reinforce the child's growing syntactic awareness. Usually, some kind of key or coding system is taught which indicates parts of speech. Separate word classes such as nouns, pronouns, verbs, and adjectives could be denoted by different coloured print or underlining. Several variations on this theme exist. One other approach has been to mark sentence structures through shapes: nouns written in a diamond, verbs in a circle, definite articles in a square, and so on. The child may be asked to compose a sentence sequence, where the grammatical relationships are given added definition through the shapes or colours. There is no particular reason why these approaches should not be tried with children who seem to be unable to grasp syntax in more natural interactive learning contexts. However, the pitfall is that the teaching of grammar becomes a pencil-and-paper exercise, not tied to direct and meaningful experience. This is, in fact, precisely what we ask many children to do in reading tests and written English exercises: make strictly grammatical decisions without any purposeful context. We have described this level of awareness of language as 'explicit'. The majority of children reach this stage of thinking about the language system as they become proficient language users at the implicit level. In other words, we would not expect children to think abstractly about the grammar of language before they have a great deal of experience in simply using it.

Finally, the principle of expectancy covers a wider range of issues than presenting written structures which reflect children's experience and competence. The worst kind of reading scheme is one which presents unidentifiable characters and lifestyles, sex-stereo-typing, cultural and racial bias, as well as unfamiliar vocabulary and syntax. Children expect stories to have a dramatic plot, emotional involvement, cohesion and resolution. Books in many reading schemes lack these aspects of real literature, and it has been said that it makes little difference whether some books are read backwards or forwards in terms of story development.

'TOP-DOWN' PROCESSES – READING FOR MEANING

There is another approach which views reading, not as a bundle of subskills, such as letter–sound decoding, but as a process which draws on higher order levels of thinking and language. According to this view, the reader approaches text by making hypotheses about what is written. The text is sampled to confirm or reject the reader's predictions. The reader looks for meaning (the right-hand side of figure 2.1) rather than letters or words, asking questions of print in order to make sense of it. A well-known proponent of this view is Smith (1978). He feels that reading is less to do with the visible marks on the page than with the knowledge and experience of language that the reader brings to the task: a natural inclination to make sense of language encounters. The evidence which is usually cited to support the 'top-down' approach, is that when children are learning to read, it is normal for mistakes to be made but that their miscues often preserve the grammar or sense of a sentence. A great deal is revealed about a child's creativity in this way (Goodman, 1976). It should be noted that 'top-down' and 'bottom-up' approaches are not necessarily incompatible, since hypotheses about text might arise from letter, sound, word, and grammar clues, together with information beyond the text, in the child's wider experience of language use.

The distinctive facet of the 'top-down' view is that it reflects much that characterises the interactive context of spoken language. Children learn to read in the same way, and using the same strategies, as they learn to speak. Both are concerned with the child's active efforts, in the company of facilitating adults, to reconstruct the system out of which meaning arises. Both suggest that children learn by experiencing something of the whole process: reading is learnt by reading books, speech through dialogue. Subskills cannot be practised or drilled, in isolation. Both assume purpose and relevance to the participants. The same conditions which help children make sense of spoken interactions with adults, also help children make sense of print.

One of the most important conditions for learning to read is the productive sharing of books between adults and children. The adult chooses books with care so that they reflect the child's concerns and experiences. For older children with less sophisticated language under control, it is important to select books with a more mature interest level, even though the language patterns may need to be less demanding. A comprehensive review of book materials appropriate to a wide range of levels and abilities has been given by Meek (1982), whilst the overall philosophy of teaching reading by reading is given practical illustration in the book edited by Moon (1985). Reading sessions need to be kept short and frequent. The focus of shared reading is to encourage children to use whatever clues they can to make sense of text. This might include an awareness of where to start in a book and in which direction to move across the pages, together with attention to headings, illustrations, and the unfolding story structure. The reading session is not an occasion to teach or correct a child. In the same way that stepping into conversation in order to elicit a correct response disrupts the flow of interaction, so the flow of meaning can be halted when adults spend too much time questioning and amending. The aim is to collaborate with the child in exploring the author's intended meaning, and not simply to achieve accurate decoding. The child is helped to question text in order to work out solutions to the linguistic puzzles presented.

Linguists sometimes refer to any stretch of language, spoken or written, as text. The strategies which the child develops in coping with text in conversation can be drawn upon in learning to read. In chapter 2 some of the text factors we identified in everyday talk include the cohesive devices which link one person's contribution to another, such as pronouns, repetition, and the sequential yoking of ideas as they develop, in terms of characters, timescale, dramatic plot. In shared reading the adult can draw the child's attention to the links which continue themes and ideas across text. When children are tackling reading materials, even at the simplest level, the most important question that adults ask is what to do when the child becomes stuck on a word. Bearing in mind that the point is to enable children to tap their own resources rather than depend on others, a number of strategies might be useful. These include inviting the child to guess from the sentence or story context, perhaps by reading onwards, or using picture clues. Predictions about what is likely to happen in a story, or in reality, can be made on a commonsense basis. Hypotheses can also be generated from textual clues, such as letter shapes and sounds. Good guesswork should always be praised, using principles such as rephrasing and expansion of what the child says, but reading errors should only be highlighted when the meaning is likely to miscarry. When that happens the child might be asked to sample the text for further clues, whilst simply supplying an important word may help to sustain the reading flow.

This approach of immersing children in authentic reading materials, as opposed to teaching by schemes, flashcards or phonic drills, is important for older children who are experiencing learning difficulties. Although the tendency might be to rehearse the subskills of reading in this group, it could be argued that these children should be given rather more help than usual to think of themselves as sources of information and to become independent, active readers. This kind of approach has been advocated recently in two publications which stemmed from a Schools Council Project entitled 'The Effective Use of Reading' (Lunzer and Gardner, 1979) and 'Learning from the Written Word' (Lunzer and Gardner, 1984). According to these authors, children often fail to grasp the function of reading. They may be led to believe, through the injudicious efforts of some teachers, that reading involves decoding from print to speech, and nothing more. To read for meaning requires a deliberate effort to make sense of what is said and to relate what is uncovered in text to what is already known. In other words, children need to be shown how to learn from their reading.

The Schools Council Project devised a series of techniques to foster reading for learning which have come to be known as 'Directed Activities Related to Texts', or 'DARTs'. Briefly, the activities are rooted in curriculum areas such as history, geography, and biology. Children test out their ideas by working in small groups. They learn how to ask the right questions of text, what to record of the information they derive, and how to check that they have the right answers. In *location* tasks, whole texts are used and children are asked to underline specific information, such as words which describe time, place or subject matter. They may be asked to set out the sequence of events in a story, to label a diagram by reading a passage, or to complete a table of information by interrogating a text. In other DARTs tasks, written material is dissected into meaning segments which children have to put into logical sequence. In *deletion* DARTs, important words or phrases are deleted from a passage and children are asked to consider how the gaps may be filled. The whole point of these exercises is to help children to become aware of the multiplicity of sources of information in reading and to use their existing capabilities more productively. This is particularly important for children who may have linguistic obstacles to overcome, such as weak vocabulary or syntax control. DARTs may help children penetrate beyond the surface features of text, and by exploiting alternative cue sources, reach a better level of understanding.

Teachers can use some of these principles for independent learning in other ways. Children can be shown how to use reference books more effectively; where to locate a name or topic in a text book using the contents page, chapter headings, or index; and how to seek out specific details by skimming or scanning. For the older child with speech and language difficulties, it is especially relevant that practice should be given at finding the way about a dictionary, timetable, newspaper, shopping catalogue, Yellow Pages, holiday brochure, gas bill, telephone directory, price list or A to Z map. One of the points made by the Bullock Report (DES, 1975) was that many youngsters are unable to read purposefully in order to follow instructions, grasp essential information, and digest and make judgements about what they find. Adults can provide the right learning conditions in which these skills are nourished. So in reading, as in the broader use of language across the curriculum, children need an awareness of effective strategies. They have to learn how to learn.

HELPING CHILDREN TO WRITE

Writing, like reading, can also be approached as one aspect of a richly interwoven tapestry of meaningful language interaction. For children with communication difficulties, writing heightens the process through which language is used to describe, convey ideas, and express reactions to experience. Everyone who writes is aware of organising, challenging, and reflecting upon one's knowledge. In schools where children are directed to write as a daily chore, the experience can be as stultifying as reading drills or language exercises may be. On the other hand, when adults create situations which demand a genuine urgency in the child to write something down, then the process may be valuable to the child's wider mastery of language.

Writing has more relevance when it is the child who takes the initiative and feels the pressure to set something in print. However, it is more typical for the teacher to decide the topic, the form of the writing and its audience. In authentic writing contexts, people write because they have feelings to express, information to give, stories to tell, requests to make, or someone to persuade. The purpose of writing is much more apparent when children are recording aspects of real-life experience, sending letters to people and receiving replies, writing notices, labels, reviews and personal journals, as opposed to filling in worksheets and coursebooks associated with some commercially available language 'laboratories'. So, the starting point for really creative writing must be that the child has something to say. For teachers working with children who have special needs in speech and language it is important that attention be paid to ways of creating conditions in which children want to write. The handing on of topics which hold meaning for the teacher is viewed less favourably than an approach which facilitates the child's own written explorations. In this respect, the principles and strategies outlined for helping oral communication and reading, the sharing of purposeful, interactive language contexts, are applied with equal weight to the fostering of writing.

In the early stages, children's ideas about the words they write often surprise adults. Children may feel that only content words which have a concrete image are real words, so that 'Mummy' and 'car' are considered to be words, but not 'if'. A word might be invested with the qualities of the object it represents, so that 'train' is thought to be a long word. This is a good example of how, even in the act of writing, children's thinking is intimately linked with its form of expression. Gradually, perhaps at about five or six years, children develop an awareness that the form language takes is separate from the objects and experiences themselves. This manipulation of words as arbitrary symbols of events reflects the child's general maturity of symbolic understanding. Writing is dependent on such development. Children have to think carefully about the language system, how a sentence is constituted and how the separate elements translate onto paper. 'Who' the writing is for is an important consideration. There are generally three distinct stages in any act of writing. First, discovering that one wishes to write by 'listening' to one's inner thoughts. Secondly, setting ideas down in print. Thirdly, reviewing what one has written, using the right words and reappraising before moving onto the next sentence. Children with speech and language problems may have difficulties at any one of these stages, which require special help.

At the first stage, then, writing requires a context which arouses in the child a genuine urge to write. An exercise set for the whole group by the teacher is unlikely to have this effect. Children may decide for themselves to record a dramatic personal experience; narrate a story; express reactions about a film, book or visit; make notes from an experiment; or write to people outside of school. All children write more purposefully on what they have recently experienced as exciting events, in stimulating stories, or through 'hands on' practical activities. Very young children can trace over a teacher's caption on a drawing. They may copy or select simple labels from a word bank, which help to fix an experience. Early written attempts should be part of an overall learning encounter: seeing, touching, feeling, talking, drawing, or making, and then encapsulating the whole in a written word or phrase. The 'Breakthrough' approach, mentioned earlier, is an effective way of relating writing to the child's interests, spoken language, and reading. Children collect a personal vocabulary store printed on small cards. A frame holds a sentence as it is constructed, which can be transferred, when the child feels it is ready, into a book. At the first stage of thinking what to write, adults can help by talking around the child's topic; drawing attention to relevant ideas, vocabulary and information; and helping children to say what they know about a subject before writing about it. This 'brainstorming' technique works because children rarely utilise all that they know.

At the second stage of writing, when ideas have to be translated into sentence patterns, children with communication difficulties are likely to require a lot of help, since this draws centrally on the child's grasp of sentence structure. At a very simple level, the teacher can discuss what the child would like to say and write a phrase or sentence using the child's own structures before the child transfers print from one place to another. Techniques such as the deletion DARTs activities used to stimulate 'top-down' skills in reading can also be helpful. The child has to select words of the appropriate grammatical class to sustain meaning in a sentence. Completion exercises and the finishing off of stem sentences make minimal demands on writing, but are the occasion for discussion and negotiation of suitable options.

Joint composition between adult and child is as important to early writing, as the active sharing of reading books. This is, in fact, one of the most useful potentials of microcomputers discussed in chapter 4, where a text-editing or story-board program allows adult and child to compose together. Openings and endings can be discussed, as well as aspects of vocabulary, sentence structure, and story sequence. If a child sticks to rigid sentence patterns, more flexible ways of presenting material can be tried. Joint writing provides an opportunity to show how punctuation is used, such as speech marks, capital letters, commas, and full stops. The adult can introduce other linguistic conventions such as time sequence (one day, after a while, just then, in the end), characterisation (she looked ..., he wore ...), and devices such as what the characters think about events in a story, flashbacks, or projections. The adult works with the child to shape, organise, and reflect upon the material.

The final stage of any act of writing involves reappraisal and revision, and yet this is rarely asked of children. Without this last stage of review, it is difficult to see how a writer can create sentences which relate to one another and make a cohesive whole. We have said that linguists refer to any stretch of language, spoken or written, as text. Children use cohesive ties in the text of spoken conversation, such as pronouns, cross-reference, and relating what is said to the topic in hand and previous utterances by repetition, very early in their oral interactions with adults. This prior experience of text features can be highlighted and developed in writing, by discussing cohesive ties, such as pronoun substitutions, with the child (Lizzie loves sweets and *her* Mum said *she* could have *some*). It is important that teachers foster the notion that writing shares many of the characteristics, functions, and intentions of speaking and reading. In both spoken language and written text the child proceeds to an explicit level of awareness of the power of language in its different forms. A collection of articles written by teachers reflecting this view of writing has been edited recently by Raban (1985).

HANDWRITING AND SPELLING

Handwriting and spelling are both skills which, to be efficient, must become automatic. We consider these 'graphological' and 'graphemic' aspects of language (see figure 2.1) to be less important than, say, the child's grasp of syntax. However, some children first earn themselves attention as having special needs because of their illegible handwriting and bizarre spelling. The latter is sometimes used as a diagnostic sign of 'dyslexia', although, as should be clear from earlier discussions, children with specific spelling or reading difficulties may simply be expressing their underlying problems in using a range of language processes. Whatever their language competencies, all children face additional obstacles if what they write is unreadable and badly spelt, since whoever reads the work is distracted from its meaning. We give here, very briefly, some practical suggestions for fostering well-formed handwriting and reliable spelling.

Children with communication difficulties need all their concentration for selecting words and sentence structures, rather than considering how letters are formed. Added problems arise if the child has poor motor co-ordination and rhythmical sense. The aim, then, is to produce a legible style which interferes minimally with the real purpose of writing. It is important for children to have good habits of posture, hand, arm, and paper position, including a tripod pen-grip, with thumb behind pen, index finger leading and middle finger supporting. Children may need to be shown individually how letter patterns are formed, using lined or squared paper as an aid together with a variety of implements. The key is short and regular practice of letter groups taken from the child's own written work. Particular movements involved in writing letter groups and combinations which are common in English can be rehearsed. It is pointless practising patterns and letter blends which are unrelated to writing itself. Many teachers feel children should be taught semi-linked letters with a joining stroke at the base, from the very beginning, whilst a looped, cursive style is outmoded and inefficient. Children may also benefit from being shown how to make pen-lifts after three or four letters, to write up to left-hand margins and to space words evenly across the page. Rote copying and repetition are less effective than sharing strategies with children, such as starting letters from the top, keeping downstrokes parallel and similar letters the same height. Ultimately, children need to be aware that handwriting for oneself requires a different quality from handwriting for more public consumption, such as job applications and form filling.

Just as there are many routes to uncover the meaning of a word as we read, so too there are several routes to encode, or spell, a word. Both spelling and reading depend on the redundancy of information in print: more cues available than are strictly necessary. Spelling errors of the kind 'wot/what', 'muny/money', 'tabul/ table' reveal that children are trying to use their knowledge of phoneme–grapheme correspondences, although English words, in the main, do not yield to such a strategy: relationships between sounds and printed letters are largely unpredictable. Another strategy might be to remember the whole visual pattern of a word. Some idea of the sentence context must be taken into account otherwise words which sound alike, such as 'hair' and 'hare', could not be distinguished. There are a number of words where it is clear that we remember the spelling on a visual-whole basis, with little interference from the letter sounds, 'yacht', 'egg', and 'who', for example. More than likely, children may attempt to copy, store and retrieve spelling patterns using a medley of strategies.

When faced with a word they are uncertain about spelling, many people feel the desire to write it down to see if it 'looks right'. What this probably indicates is that words are more easily remembered as visual patterns. Research evidence suggests (Marsh et al., 1980) that whilst children start out by using letter–sound correspondences in order to spell, a shift in strategies occurs. Eventually, proficient spellers build up a visual store of word patterns which can be retrieved automatically or by analogy (bicycle/recycle). The fact that deaf children have few spelling problems (Webster, 1986a) suggests that it is the visual rather than the sound similarities which are significant. There are some important principles for the teaching of spelling to be noted. Firstly, words should be selected which the child wishes to use. Like many aspects of language skill addressed in this book, spelling is least efficiently learned in rote fashion, from lists or cards, without a genuine context or purpose. Three or four indispensable and frequently occurring words should be high-lighted in a child's written work, rather than marking every error. Inserting letters in a word which is wrong is poor practice. When a child attempts spelling corrections, a reliable procedure is to write the word for the child, ask the child to read it, cover it over, and then see if the child can reproduce it from memory. Using this method the child learns, not by copying letter-for-letter, but in visual wholes. Extensions of this work include identifying word families of similar internal structure (require, bequest, request). Independence in spelling implies that the child has the reference skills to be able to confirm the spelling of a word in a dictionary.

PARENTS AND THE INTERVENTION PROCESS

Throughout this book we have stressed the important role which parents play in their children's developmental progress, and this is no less true of children with special needs. Many parents do have points of their own to make, and deserve adequate explanations and advice which can be implemented realistically at home. There is a wealth of evidence to suggest that the spontaneous skills of parents as language facilitators provide the key to fostering communication when children experience difficulties. However, we do know that some children evoke less nurturing styles of interaction from adults, and provide fewer cues for adults to respond to. Social interactions which are linguistically unproductive may lead to emotionally charged relationships, anxiety, and guilt. This is especially marked when parents themselves experienced communication problems as children, and possibly have negative recollections of school.

Parental involvement begins with their close and continual involvement with professionals at the time any assessments, recommendations and reviews are made. To some extent the rights of parents, both informal and formal, are set down in the 1981 Education Act and the guidance to local authorities which accompanies it. Apart from general advice about professionals being open and honest with parents, schools have particular responsibilities for careful record keeping and involving parents in reviews and when any changes are required. Within certain strictures parents can request a full multi-professional assessment of their child's needs, and a full review is mandatory at 13 years in order to decide future options up to the age of 18 years or so. Parents can be asked to participate in the setting of realistic teaching objectives and it is essential, at points of transfer such as junior to secondary school, that parents are helped to make informed decisions. That may, in many instances, require visits to be made to different kinds of school settings.

Parents, as well as children, can be included in the wider community of the school, in many ways. Open days, festival occasions, sports galas, concerts, PTA meetings, jumble sales, newsletters, and fund-raising events should automatically include the parents of children with special needs, even where children spend only part of the time in mainstream. It is particularly helpful when parents live some distance away from a specially-resourced school, that there is frequent contact between school staff and home, with details such as telephone extension numbers and the best times of which days to contact each other. At the beginning of this chapter some suggestions were made as to how parents can be directly involved in the classroom, once roles have been clearly defined. Similarly, the home–school book is one means of parents and teachers keeping each other in touch with important events.

As a final comment on language intervention, many of the strategies outlined here for productive interaction between adults and children, although derived from natural learning contexts, can, in turn, be handed back to parents to use at home, especially where parents have lost confidence in their own abilities and need to be reassured. Strategies for gaining the child's attention; encouraging symbolic play; centring talk upon a shared experience; sustaining conversation; expanding and clarifying what the child intends to say; allowing the child time to respond; the issue of control and initiative; questioning; sharing books; and the place of direct teaching techniques: all these aspects are important in the home context too. Inevitably, this widens the responsibility of teachers and professionals, since their advice has to stand up to the rigours of parental trial and feedback, which is perhaps not a bad thing.

An overview for the ordinary teacher

We have set out in this book to help professionals, particularly teachers, who want to know more about the special needs of children with speech and language difficulties in the ordinary school. Hopefully, too, those with special responsibility for children with communication difficulties, together with other support agencies, such as remedial staff, speech therapists, and educational psychologists, will have found the book useful. No practical guide, however well designed or illustrated, can fulfil its purpose or convince its audience, without a firm theoretical grounding. The first major aim has been to provide a clear conceptual model of normal speech and language development, within a context of social interaction. The stance we have adopted is that unless we can describe, with some confidence, how the majority of children proceed from being language novice to language expert, then our explanations of how development can go awry will be more than hesitant.

Language is so heavily interwoven with many aspects of normal psychological development that it should not require an exclusive set of rules to describe how it unfolds. In fact the strategies children adopt for learning to communicate are no different from any other kind of learning. We accept that all children have a potential to learn. Children often appear to be impelled to discover more about their environments. From the earliest stages, children actively test out and explore their surroundings, piecing together the evidence of their experience. Making sense of the world requires an ability to organise and categorise objects and events. Language imposes its own kind of grid on the child's perceptions and thinking, at the same time that the child's encounters make demands upon the language system, in order to reflect experience. We place the child centrally in the learning process, not as a passive assimilator of information, but as a scientist forming hypotheses about the way things work and applying the rules which are generated to new situations. Adults have a crucial role to play: they seem to be superbly proficient in providing just the right kind of feedback to the learner. In the ordinary course of events adults provide the stimulus and opportunity for linguistic interaction to occur, in order to facilitate the child's learning.

In describing the course of language development we have outlined the traditional levels of structure: sounds, grammar, and semantics. A stage approach to these different aspects provides a series of bench-marks which enable us to judge the relative maturity of children when compared with each other. This approach to language leaves unanswered the intriguing question of *how* the child learns. The recent evidence which we have (Snow and Ferguson, 1977; Tizard and Hughes, 1984; Wells, 1981) suggests that the key to learning is to be found in conversational interaction. We have highlighted a range of strategies which parents spontaneously use in talking with their children which serve to engage the child in interaction; improve the child's access to the language system by simplifying and clarifying what is said; negotiate meanings with the child in relation to a shared context; and sustain the child's involvement as a language partner. Meaning and purpose are axiomatic. Language is, in a sense, a by-product of shared, purposeful activity. For that reason, the power of language for the child is the range of social and intellectual functions it serves.

The second major aim of this book has been to give teachers a clear view of how language development might go astray, the kind of difficulties encountered in schools, and the likely numbers of children involved. It will be apparent that the field of language difficulty covers a very wide range of factors, from relatively minor speech-articulation problems to severe sensory handicaps. Normal language development depends on intact senses, motor skills, intelligence, and a social environment in which the child's emotional needs are nourished. If any one of these dimensions is disturbed, it is likely that the pattern of language development will also be affected. In chapter 3, a brief examination was made of the more obvious factors known to be involved in speech and language difficulties, such as vision and hearing. We have deliberately avoided the grouping together of children under diagnostic categories, such as 'aphasic', preferring to concentrate on the parameters which can be used to describe the particular strengths and weaknesses of individuals. We have not neglected the likely possibility that communication difficulties themselves lead to disturbances in the social and emotional well-being of families and children. We can only understand the full implications of a child's communication difficulties by observing transactions between the child and peers, family, or learning environment.

Teachers not only need to know how development proceeds and how it might go wrong; they also need to be able to identify potential problems and take steps to seek help. Some guidelines based on a collective knowledge of the behaviour of typical children are given. Commercially available tests have their place in identifying the special language needs of a particular child, and it is hoped that the book has provided a working perspective which allows teachers to judge for themselves the merit of insights gained from commercial packages. However, the teacher's best insights will stem from an understanding of the skills that are appropriate at a given age. The teacher has a range of responsibilities in terms of identifying and appraising children's special needs, some of which are spelled out in the 1981 Education Act and the advice to local education authorities which accompanied it. In the 'informal' stages described under this legislation, it is important that teachers are careful in their screening, monitoring, and record keeping about children, and in communicating any concerns to parents and supporting professionals. In the 'formal' stages, the teacher's observations are very important in shaping a child's profile of needs and the likely response which is made to meet them. In the end it is largely left to the teacher to ask for more help, to build satisfactory working links with outside professionals, to make relationships with parents, and to carry on with the day-to-day business of the classroom.

What, then, can teachers do to help children with speech and language difficulties in their classrooms? Two reactions are commonplace. First, to bombard a child with remedial teaching and 'special' materials. Secondly, for teachers to feel anxious about their own competence to help. It is unfortunately the case that some children compound their own learning difficulties by evoking styles of behaviour in adults which are less nurturing than they would otherwise be. The question that has to be asked at that point is 'What needs to be done differently, if anything?' It is our considered view that all children have a disposition to learn, in the right conditions. This is no less true of children affected by handicapping factors. It simply means that greater attention has to be paid to the context in which the child learns. It could be argued that it is precisely the child who has difficulties in communicating who is most in need of the kind of interactive experiences which characterise normal adult–child encounters and which provide the well-tailored evidence from which children learn.

THE STRENGTHS OF THE ORDINARY TEACHER

An underlying theme of this book is that opportunities for using language are inherent in the day-to-day experiences across the curriculum and in the informal encounters in school. Paradoxically, the more that the focus shifts towards communication as an isolated end in itself the less likely it is to occur. One of the inevitable hazards of trying to make formal assessments of children's speech and language is that to do so changes the nature of the communicative experience for both adult and child in a way which is likely to be unproductive. For that reason, formal tests must have a subsidiary role of supporting the insights of the teacher. There are similar dangers in assuming that speech and language forms can be taught directly, through commercial programmes or set-pieces. Again, teachers may wish to select materials which sustain and reinforce their own particular methodology. However, we have argued that the teacher's best efforts should be aimed at optimising conditions for learning. The bedrock of successful intervention is an awareness of how adults can modify their interactions with children in order to foster language and thinking. Teachers must be led towards a critical self-awareness and self-evaluation of the effects of their language interventions on others. But the medium, or culture, for language acquisition is the classroom context and curriculum. The aware teacher will seize the opportunities which arise naturally from the contexts in which language is used as an integral component of the learning experience.

All teachers possess qualities of practice which enable children to learn more efficiently, and we can highlight those particular strengths which meet the needs of children with communication difficulties. In the early stages particularly, predictable patterns for the day and consistent learning routines help children feel secure and comfortable. A clear sense of purpose is fostered if children know that work will be looked at; a promised story read; a time set aside regularly to talk about a reading book; and any sanctions cautioned, followed through. The basis of good practice is consistency in what teachers say and do. Good teachers provide clear aims and objectives in their work, both for themselves and for children to follow. In the classroom, they give clear expectations regarding assignments and the timescale within which tasks should be completed. Anticipated behaviour, for example, on an outing, is spelled out. Children are instructed how to ask for help, move about the room, address others. Clear starting and stopping points are given, so that children know when to move on from one topic to another. Feedback is always provided to let children know how well they have done. Children's progress is discussed openly with those concerned.

In a well-organised classroom environment the timetable has balance so that children are not working at formal tasks continuously, spending all morning listening; or, as can happen, sitting watching TV programmes in one subject area after another. A varied diet, with work in a small group interspersed with larger class presentations, perhaps for a story, together with contrasting ways of presenting information, all help. 'Hands-on' experience brings a subject alive. Children with limited attention and poor auditory skills do not thrive in a mayhem of distracting stimulation. All children enjoy a workmanlike atmosphere. Well-arranged equipment, ordered storage, clear labelling, and the attractive display of books, work, and project materials, set models of behaviour. In many respects, then, what turns out to be helpful for children with special needs in speech and language can be applied to the majority.

WHAT DO TEACHERS NEED TO DO DIFFERENTLY?

Adults often ask what should be tackled differently, when a child presents communication difficulties. Nothing that we have said in this book proposes a radical change in teaching styles or curriculum content. What we have argued for is an enhancement of those features of adult responsiveness and good teaching practice that facilitate meaning-oriented, collaborative learning. In conversation, which is the heart of the language acquisition process, the intention should be to communicate. Adults spontaneously achieve this with young children by gaining attention; sharing a focus of interest; agreeing a topic of conversation; clarifying what is said through paraphrase, repetition, and clear pronunciation; relating what is said to previous utterances; pitching language structurally just beyond the child's; allowing the child initiative and time to respond; and by giving 'social oil' and personal contributions. These strategies were discussed in some detail in chapter 5.

Bearing these principles in mind, teachers should be able to work out how they might respond when faced with any child with a speech or language difficulty. Let us take one example – a child with a stammer. The adult's strategy should be to aim for meaning. Gestures, pointing, and body language may help. The adult should try to reflect what the child is thinking or feeling, at the appropriate level. The child may be anxious and expect embarrassment. Anxiety can be reduced by calm reactions, avoiding hurrying the child, and, when the conversational turn is handed over, responding by putting the child's intended meaning into words. Indeed, the adult can reflect a child's communicative purpose, even though the child has said nothing: 'You're upset because you've missed your dinner, are you?' 'You're having trouble with that puzzle, aren't you?' What the adult interprets from the social context must always, of course, be open to negotiation with the child.

In the wider scope of language use, teachers need to be aware of the copious opportunities for language enrichment which arise intrinsically from the curriculum. The aware teacher is an opportunist, seizing openings in humanities, art, PE, music, and dance, together with formal areas of the curriculum to foster listening, questioning, turn-taking, and aspects of language use. Language as a tool for learning other things is also acquired and developed by being put to use. A good teacher marks out a topic of interest; catches and inspires children's sense of discovery; and, by shaping the enquiry, helps children to work over their experience productively. Essentially, the direction in which the learning process moves is towards the children's active independence as learners, aware of how to go about their own study. This emphasis applies to a wide variety of learning contexts, including speech and language, reading, spelling, and writing. The child's own initiatives are fostered, in a meaning-oriented partnership, where the child can test out hypotheses against experience.

WHAT SHOULD TEACHERS AVOID?

During the course of this book we have given numerous examples of what appear to be less facilitative ways of approaching children in close language encounters, and in the classroom context. Anything that blocks the engagement of children in interaction will be unhelpful to those with communication needs. For that reason, classroom management should be well considered so that adults are available for some of the time to work closely with individuals. Inevitably, if teaching is based solely on whole-class presentations with few opportunities for interaction, then those opportunities may not be taken up at all by the children who would benefit most. A dominating, controlling, and managerial style may also be inhibiting to some children. Where children are not allowed to take the initiative, where the adult chooses topics and themes, and where the teacher tends to over-question, the child may become guarded. Test questions such as 'What colour are your shoes?' may be viewed by the child as cross-examination. Display questions are much less facilitative than genuine enquiries which solicit the child's views, ideas, and preferences: 'Is that your favourite colour?' Similarly, listening to what children have to say half-heartedly whilst doing something else, finishing off what the child is trying to say, and not allowing time to respond, are all inhibitory. The way in which an adult talks to children has a determining effect on how forthcoming they are as participants.

In our view there are good reasons to avoid correcting, enforced imitation of sentence models, and the direct teaching of parts of language. Whilst direct teaching techniques may have their place in some clinical settings or as backup work, we are unconvinced of the need to look beyond the genuine opportunities for language use which arise spontaneously in school. We apply the same logic to the teaching of reading or writing through drills and exercises. The opinion we hold is that reading is best taught through reading, writing through writing, and language through real communication. Some commonsense is necessary. In modelling, for example, there is a world of difference between the teacher who gives this advice to a child: 'It might be better if you said "Please may I join in the game?"', and the teacher who insists that a correct sentence is repeated: 'Say "Nobody likes me."' Perhaps the very worst example of an elicitation technique is where the whole of a group of children is asked to chant in unison. The misconceptions of children taught 'The Lord's Prayer' in this way survive into adulthood.

Children know when they are being prompted into talking for talking's sake, and when they are being patronised or bribed. Adult responsiveness means entering conversation as equal partners with children, not being condescending or syrupy-sweet. When teachers are genuine with children, explaining their thinking and the reasons for their plans, then children feel valued and have a sense of self-esteem, even though they may have severe learning obstacles to face. Incentives for speaking, such as rewarding a child with a toy, or producing a drink only when asked properly, should be used with care. Almost all that we have said implies that language behaviour is not an object in its own right to be manipulated. Wherever possible the impulse to use language should arise essentially from the function it serves.

A SUMMARY OF GOOD PRACTICE FOR HELPING COMMUNICATION

The developmental evidence which has guided our thinking suggests a number of important learning principles, not specific to language, which underpin good practice for enabling communication in children with special needs.

The starting point should be where the child is

All good teaching starts from where the learner is and moves outwards. Careful observation, using a developmental framework, will reveal what the child can and cannot do, in different skill areas. Teaching objectives and the sequence of learning steps should be set down clearly. Learning tasks must take into account the child's

experience and level of awareness, building on existing competence. Account should be taken of topics the child initiates, both in
conversation and in the classroom.

Content must be meaningful

In conversation children and adults do not talk about nothing; they
discuss things of mutual concern embedded in joint activity. The
content of learning must matter. Children are impelled to use
language in situations which are meaningful to themselves and
their lives. Remote content will produce little momentum. This is an
important guiding principle when stories, materials, and books are
chosen, and when classroom activities are planned. Schools must be
wary of presenting an alien culture to children and families.

Function and purpose must be clear

Language serves a wide range of functions: expressing feelings and
needs, maintaining social contact, controlling others, escaping into
fantasy, as well as being a tool for learning and thinking. The
teacher should seize the opportunities which arise for using
language in different ways in different areas of the curriculum.
Children gain a sense of purpose when they know the function of a
learning exercise and how language is to be put to use.

Children learn through interaction

Children learn language in a context of social interaction. Mere
exposure to the forms of language is inadequate. Adults collaborate
with children, using a range of strategies in order to communicate.
Interaction, whereby the adult negotiates meaning with the child, is
important for reading and for classwork. There must be opportunities for discussion and planning between peers, and between adult
and child.

Children are active explorers not passive assimilators

We place the child centrally in the learning process, actively using
the evidence which language encounters provide, in order to make
sense of the language system. Adults provide the learning
conditions in which children can test out their hypotheses. In
reading and across the curriculum, children should be encouraged
to question, seek out rules and reconstruct their own models of how
the world works.

Adults should be responsive

Adults vary in their responsiveness. Language flourishes when adults respond by listening to what the child has to say; expanding, paraphrasing, and clarifying the child's intended meaning; sustaining the child's involvement with social oil; handing conversation back to the child, and allowing time for reply. It is the adult's input which provides the linguistic evidence from which children learn.

Language is least effectively learnt through direct teaching

The teacher's efforts are best directed towards the conditions within which learning takes place. When adults try to teach language directly the focus of communication moves from the sharing of meaning towards the form of language. Language cannot be dispensed bit-by-bit from a programme without a purposeful social context. When children are put in the position of passive respondent to the adult's demands, learning is sterotyped. When language drills and kits are used, the interactive experience is less nurturing.

The curriculum is a fund for language use

Language is both system and resource. It is a means to learn other things, as well as being learnt through use. Language enrichment opportunities are intrinsic throughout the curriculum. The aware teacher seizes opportunities in all subject areas, formal and informal, in order to foster language enquiry. Since language is such an integral part of almost all social and intellectual experience, it is misguided to discuss it, or teach it, as a subject set apart.

The same principles for helping spoken language apply to literacy

What children learn in their encounters with spoken language is later applied to reading and writing. Children approach print with the same expectations, learning styles, and intentions that characterise their experience of oral communication. Learning to read and write should be approached as a meaning-oriented, collaborative partnership, facilitated by social interaction. Reading for meaning and writing for a purpose, harness the child's natural strengths of enquiry in just the same way that spoken dialogue does.

Work should be in partnership

Perhaps the most important principle has been left to the last. All professionals have a responsibility to share information, ideas and effective strategies. Teachers need to work closely with all those concerned and should not be afraid to ask for help and advice if they feel unsupported, or are concerned about a child's progress. Working partnerships with families are paramount if there is to be continuity between what happens at home and in school. After all, the often unacknowledged language 'experts' are the children and parents themselves.

Appendix 1 Developmental screening checklists for speech and language difficulties in young children

HEALTH VISITOR SCREENING AT TWO YEARS

In the majority of two-year-olds useful language is developing out of day-to-day activities and exploratory play. Potential problems may be identified in children who fail four out of ten items.

Language Behaviour	Examples
1. Put two or more words together to express feelings, make statements.	'Want juice', 'Daddy gone'
2. Indicate plurals	'Find Mummy shoes', 'Lot cars'
3. Ask simple content questions.	'What that?', 'Doing Mummy?'
4. Accompany play and reflect experience with verbal commentary.	'All broke', 'Teddy drink'
5. Show and name body parts on request.	hair, eyes, tummy
6. Give name in response to questions.	
7. Follow a two-part command.	'Put the paper in the bin', 'Give the shoe to baby'
8. Point to familiar objects on request.	cup, chair, door, ball
9. Can be distracted from a forbidden object to another attraction.	
10. Join in nursery rhymes, jingles and songs.	

NURSERY SCREENING AT THREE AND A HALF YEARS

Children have normally begun to externalise language by this age: they 'think' and 'work' out loud. Teachers should be concerned about children who fail four or more items and should seek further advice.

Language Behaviour	*Examples*
1. Use four to five word sentences intelligible to most people.	'He's coming in the door', 'Mummy's gone to grandma's'
2. Ask what, where, who questions.	
3. Can select and describe objects by use.	'Which do we eat with?', 'You put it on your head'
4. Change word order for questions.	'Can I watch TV?'
5. Use most prepositions and pronouns appropriately.	'Daddy's up the ladder', 'She's jumping on my castle'
6. Participate in simple conversations: give and receive.	
7. Can recount past events, remember and describe routines.	'My Daddy did take us to Thorpe Park'
8. Respond appropriately to sentences including colour, size, and quantity.	'Give me the big red ball'
9. Approach adults and peers with requests for permission, explanation, or justification.	'Why are we going?'
10. Use comparative forms.	'longest', 'hotter', 'smaller'

TEACHER SCREENING AT FIVE YEARS

Language has usually reached a level of competence which forms the basis for reasoning, imagining, and self-expression beyond the immediate context. Four or more failures should signal concern and referral for professional advice.

Language Behaviour	*Examples*
1. Language is generally fluent and grammatical with minor speech immaturities.	
2. Explain the meaning of simple words, ask meaning of abstract words.	'Tired's when you go to bed' 'What's mysterious?'
3. Listen to or tell a familiar story without the aid of picture clues.	
4. Enjoy verbal humour and riddles.	'Knock, knock, who's there?'
5. Respond appropriately to complex directions without the need to follow other children's leads.	'When you've finished your picture, put all your books on my table'
6. Maintain attention on a task whilst listening to adult instructions.	
7. Attempt to write own first name and draw a recognisable man/woman.	
8. Use language to reason out situations or problems.	'You have to stay near your Mum or you may get lost'
9. Use complex structures with co-ordinated or embedded sentence patterns.	'I used some of the new pens you gave me to make a picture for you'
10. Enjoy picture books, have a growing sight vocabulary.	

Appendix 2 Further information sources

HELPING ORGANISATIONS

1. AFASIC (Association for All Speech-Impaired Children),
   347 Central Markets,
   Smithfield,
   London. EC1A 9NH
   Campaigns for specialised provision and publicises the needs of children with language difficulties.

2. British Dyslexia Association,
   Church Lane,
   Peppard,
   Henley,
   Oxon. RG9 5JN
   Represents some 70 local associations which give advice on the teaching and assessment of children with specific learning disabilities.

3. CLAPA (Cleft Lip and Palate Association),
   1 Eastwood Gardens,
   Kenton,
   Newcastle-upon-Tyne. NE3 3DQ
   Primarily supports self-help groups for parents, together with research and publicity.

4. College of Speech Therapists,
   Harold Poster House,
   6 Lechmere Road,
   London. NW2 5BU
   The professional organisation for speech therapists, which publishes journals, information leaflets and a directory of members.

5. ICAA (Invalid Children's Aid Association),
   126 Buckingham Palace Road,
   London. SW1W 9SB

Provides teaching resources for children with speech and language disorders; has four residential special schools, a social work and information service.

6. NATLIC (National Association of Teachers of Language Impaired Children),
2 Vernon Close,
St Peter's Field,
Martley,
Worcs. WR6 6QX
Promotes professional awareness of needs of language-impaired children amongst teachers, therapists and other professionals, encourages effective practice and disseminates information.

7. VOCAL (Voluntary Organisations Communication and Language),
336 Brixton Road,
London. SW9 7AA
Represents a number of charities involved in supporting, promoting and funding professionals and families involved with communication disabilities.

8. NDCS (National Deaf Children's Society),
45 Hereford Road,
London. W2 5AH
Promotes education, interests, and public awareness of special needs of deaf children; represents 140 regions and branches offering self-help support; provides information service through its education officer.

JOURNALS

Child Language Teaching and Therapy, edited by D. Crystal, published by Edward Arnold, London

The editorial policy of this journal is to raise practical issues relevant to the teaching of children with a wide range of language difficulties, including communication problems arising from deafness, emotional problems, physical or learning handicaps, and English as a second language. Papers are published on assessment, teaching techniques, and professional roles. This is an interdisciplinary journal which avoids very specialised or technical material and is accessible to all those professionally involved and who wish to keep up to date.

British Journal of Disorders of Communication, edited by R. Lesser, published by the College of Speech Therapists

This journal covers research aspects in any area of concern to speech therapists including audiology, phonetics, neurology, education, and child psychology. Selected articles may be useful to teachers, although this is a fairly specialised journal.

Journal of Child Language, edited by A. Cruttenden, published by Cambridge University Press

This journal publishes research material on all aspects of language behaviour in children, including normal and atypical development. Studies of literacy, therapy and remedial education are also included, reflecting the growing edge of the scientific study of child language acquisition.

Journal of Speech and Hearing Disorder, edited by L. B. Leonard, published by the American Speech–Language–Hearing Association

Articles are published relating to the nature and treatment of disordered speech, hearing, and language, as well as professional issues, such as the organisation and evaluation of intervention programmes. It has a clinical, rather than a purely research focus, and provides a useful update on current professional practice, but is academically demanding.

RELATED BOOKS

Cook, V. J. (1979) *Young Children and Language* London, Edward Arnold.

This is a good introductory book, written in an accessible style. It describes the development of language in young children and the functions this serves in play, thinking, and reasoning, and in early literacy. Most useful, perhaps, for parents, it gives some very basic suggestions for helping children and some initial answers to questions like 'What should I do with a child who does not speak in a playgroup?'

Crystal, D. (1980) *Introduction to Language Pathology* London, Edward Arnold.

The author's aim in this book has been to provide a general but informative view of language disability for students in professional training. The strength of the text is the concise explanations of terminology, language models, and the interdisciplinary overlaps which exist in the therapeutic field. This is a fairly demanding book, useful as a reference text for teachers, although its scope does not extend to practical intervention in the classroom.

de Villiers, J. G. and de Villiers, P. A. (1978) *Language Acquisition* **Cambridge, Massachusetts, Harvard University Press.**

In this clearly written and authoritative book, the authors provide a lively account of children's acquisition of sounds, meaning, and syntax. The treatment is broad and thorough, dealing with issues such as the genetic predisposition to learn language in humans, critical periods, and language in developmentally-disabled children. Research is summarised succinctly with plenty of practical examples, though the focus is not an educationalist's one.

Garvey, C. (1984) *Children's Talk* **London, Fontana Paperbacks.**

This book describes how young children interact with each other in social situations using newly acquired verbal skills to achieve particular goals, such as gaining the upper hand, saying 'No', and making requests. A lot of the data comes from recordings of pairs of children in a play context. This is a very readable account of an integrated approach to language as social interaction.

Hastings, P. and Hayes, B. (1981) *Encouraging Language Development* **Beckenham, Croom Helm.**

This is a short volume (68 pages) in a series of books directed at professionals and parents, intended to share good practice. The text is well-illustrated with photographs and covers a wide area: hearing loss, mental retardation, behaviour difficulties. It is a good, first introduction to the field with simple suggestions about play, attention, talking to children, identifying problems, and encouraging early language stages. It lacks a theoretical framework and is a little superficial. Classroom problems are not addressed and the book will have greatest appeal to parents.

Bloom, L. and Lahey, M. (1978) *Language Development and Language Disorders* **London, John Wiley and Sons.**

An American text, this is a comprehensive source book with a great deal of information about normal and atypical language development. Teachers may find there is too much technical content, but it does address assessment issues, the setting of teaching goals, and intervention techniques.

Browning, E. (1972) *I Can't See What You're Saying* **London, Paul Elek Books.**

This is a personal account by the mother of an 'asphasic' child which describes the problems parents sometimes face in dealing with professionals, in reaching understanding of their child's problems, and in discovering strategies to circumvent the minutiae of day-to-day obstacles which appear when a child's understanding and use of language is impaired.

References

Ainscow, M., and Tweddle, D. M. (1979) *Preventing Classroom Failure: an Objectives Approach*, London: Wiley and Sons.

Anderson, E. M., and Spain, B. (1977) *The Child with Spina Bifida*, London: Methuen.

Anderson, L. M., Evertson, C. M., and Emmer, E. T. (1980) Dimensions in classroom management derived from recent research. *Journal of Curriculum Studies* **12** (4), pp. 343–356.

Anthony, A., Bogle, D., Ingram, T. T. S., and McIsaac, M. W. (1971) *The Edinburgh Articulation Test*, Edinburgh: Livingstone.

Barnes, S. B., Gutfreund, M., Satterly, D. J., and Wells, C. G. (1983) Characteristics of adult speech which predict children's language development. *Journal of Child Language* **10**, pp. 65–84.

Bax, M., Hart, H., and Jenkins, S. (1983) The behaviour, development and health of the young child: implications for care. *British Medical Journal* **286**, pp. 1793–1796.

Bernstein, B. (1965) 'A socio-linguistic approach to social learning' in J. Gould (ed.) *Penguin Survey of the Social Sciences*, Harmondsworth: Penguin.

Bernstein, B. (ed.) (1973) *Class, Codes and Control. Vol 2: Applied Studies Towards a Sociology of Language*, London: Routledge and Kegan Paul.

Beveridge, M. (ed.) (1982) *Children Thinking through Language*, London: Edward Arnold.

Bishop, D. V. M. (1983) *Test for Reception of Grammar*, London: Medical Research Council.

Blank, M. (1985) 'Classroom discourse: the neglected topic of the topic' in M. M. Clark (ed.) *Helping Communication in Early Education*, Birmingham: University of Birmingham, Educational Review Occasional Publications (11), pp. 13–20.

Brown, R. (1977) 'Introduction' in C. E. Snow and C. A. Ferguson (eds) *Talking to Children*, Cambridge: Cambridge University Press.

Bruner, J. S. (1975) The ontogenesis of speech acts. *Journal of Child Language* **2**, pp. 1–19.

Bryant, P., and Bradley, L. (1985) *Children's Reading Problems*, Oxford: Blackwell.

Calnan, M., and Richardson, K. (1976) Speech problems in a national survey. *Child: Care, Health and Development* **2** (4), pp. 181–202.

Carrow, E. (1973) *Test for Auditory Comprehension of Language*, Boston, Massachusetts: Teaching Resources Corporation.

Chapman, E. K. (1978) *Visually Handicapped Children and Young People*, London: Routledge and Kegan Paul.

Chapman, E., and Stone, J. (forthcoming) *Visual Handicaps in the Classroom*, London: Cassell.

Chazan, M., Laing, A. F., Bailey, M. S., and Jones, G. (1980) *Some of Our Children: the Early Education of Children with Special Needs*, London: Open Books.

Clark, H. H., and Clark, E. V. (1977) *Psychology and Language: An Introduction to Psycholinguistics*, New York: Harcourt Brace Jovanovich.

Clark, M. M. (1976) *Young Fluent Readers*, London: Heinemann.

Conrad, R. (1979) *The Deaf School Child*, London: Harper and Row.

Cooke, J., and Williams, D. (1985) *Working with Children's Language*, Buckingham: Winslow Press.

Cooper, J., Moodley, M., and Reynell, J. (1978) *Helping Language Development: A Developmental Programme for Children with Early Language Handicaps*, London: Edward Arnold.

Crystal, D. (1976) *Child Language, Learning and Linguistics*, London: Edward Arnold.

Crystal, D. (1984) *Language Handicap in Children*, Stratford-upon-Avon: National Council for Special Education.

Crystal, D., Fletcher, P., and Garman, M. (1976) *The Grammatical Analysis of Language Disability*, London: Edward Arnold.

Cummins, J. (1984) *Bilingualism and Special Education: Issues in Assessment and Pedagogy*, Clevedon: Multilingual Matters.

Dale, P. S. (1976) *Language Development: Structure and Function* 2nd edn, New York: Holt, Rinehart and Winston.

Davie, R., Butler, N., and Goldstein, H. (1972) *From Birth to Seven*, London: Longman.

DES (1967) *Children and Their Primary Schools* (The Plowden Report), London: HMSO.

DES (1972) *Speech Therapy Services* (The Quirk Report), London: HMSO.

DES (1975) *A Language for Life* (The Bullock Report), London: HMSO.

DES (1978) *Primary Education in England*, London: HMSO.

DES (1978) *Special Educational Needs* (The Warnock Report), London: HMSO.

DES (1985) *Education for All* (The Swann Report), London: HMSO.

Devereux, K. (1981) *Understanding Learning Difficulties*, Milton Keynes: Open University Press.

de Villiers, J. G., and de Villiers, P. A. (1979) *Early Language*, London: Open Books.

Deykin, E. Y., and MacMahon, B. (1979) The incidence of seizures among children with autistic symptoms. *American Journal of Psychiatry* **136**, pp. 1310–1312.

Dodd, B. (1976) The phonological systems of deaf children. *Journal of Speech and Hearing Disorders* **41**, pp. 185–198.

Donaldson, M. (1978) *Children's Minds*, London: Fontana.

Dowling, M. (1980) *Early Projects*, London: Longman.

Downing, J., Ayers, D., and Schaefer, B. (1983) *Linguistic Awareness in Reading Readiness Test*, Windsor: NFER-Nelson.

Downs, M. P. (1977) 'The expanding imperatives of early identification' in F. Bess (ed.) *Childhood Deafness: Causation, Assessment and Management*, New York: Grune and Stratton, pp. 95–106.
Dunn, L. M., Dunn, L. M., and Whetton, C. (1981) *British Picture Vocabulary Scales*, Windsor: NFER-Nelson.

Edwards, A. D. (1976) *Language in Culture and Class*, London: Heinemann.
Edwards, J. R. (1979) *Language and Disadvantage*, London: Edward Arnold.
Engelmann, S., and Osborn, J. (1976) *DISTAR Language 1* 2nd edn, Science Research Association.

Ferrier, L. J. (1978) 'Some observations of error in context' in N. Waterson and C. E. Snow (eds) *The Development of Communication*, Chichester: Wiley.
Fundudis, T., Kolvin, I., and Garside, R. (eds) (1979) *Speech Retarded and Deaf Children: Their Psychological Development*, London: Academic Press.
Furth, H. G. (1966) *Thinking Without Language*, New York: Free Press.

Gagné, R. M. (1977) *The Conditions of Learning* 3rd edn, New York: Holt, Rinehart and Winston.
Garvey, C. (1977) *Play*, London: Fontana.
Gillham, B. (1979) *The First Words Language Programme*, London: George Allen and Unwin, *and* Beaconsfield: Beaconsfield Publishers.
Gillham, B. (1983) *Two Words Together*, London: George Allen and Unwin.
Gittelman, R., and Feingold, I. (1983) Children with reading disorders: I. efficacy of reading remediation. *Journal of Child Psychology and Psychiatry* **24**, pp. 167–191.
Goodman, K. S. (1976) 'Reading: a psycholinguistic guessing game', in H. Singer and R. Ruddell (eds) *Theoretical Models and Processes of Reading* 2nd edn, Newark, Delaware: International Reading Association.
Graham, N. (1980) 'Memory constraints in language deficiency' in F. M. Jones (ed.) *Language Disability in Children*, Lancaster: MTP Press.
Gregory, S. (1983) 'The development of communication skills in young deaf children: Delayed or deviant?' Paper presented to the Child Language Seminar, University of Strathclyde, March 1983.
Gregory, S., and Mogford, K. (1981) 'Early language development in deaf children' in B. Woll, J. Kyle, and M. Deuchar (eds) *Perspectives in British Sign Language and Deafness*, London: Croom Helm.

Halliday, M. A. K. (1975) *Learning how to Mean – Explorations in the Development of Language*, London: Edward Arnold.
Harris, J. (1984) Early language intervention programmes: An update. *Association for Child Psychology and Psychiatry Newsletter* **6** (2), pp. 2–21.
Hutt, E. (1986) *Teaching Language-Disordered Children: A Structured Curriculum*, London: Edward Arnold.

Ingram, D. (1976) *Phonological Disability in Children. Studies in Language Disability and Remediation II*, London: Edward Arnold.

Ingram, T. T. S. (1963) 'Report of the Dysphasia Sub-committee of the Scottish Paediatric Society' (mimeograph).

Jeffree, D. M., and McConkey, R. (1976) *Let Me Speak*, London: Souvenir Press.
Jeffree, D. M., McConkey, R., and Hewson, S. (1977) *Let Me Play*, London: Souvenir Press.

Karmiloff-Smith, A. (1978) 'The interplay between syntax, semantics and phonology in language processes' in R. N. Campbell and P. T. Smith (eds) *Recent Advances in the Psychology of Language*, New York: Plenum Press.
Karnes, M. (1977) *Goal Oriented Activities for Learning – Levels 1 and 2*, Springfield, Massachusetts: Milton Bradley.
Kirk, S. A., McCarthy, J. J., and Kirk, W. D. (1968) *Illinois Test of Psycholinguistic Abilities* Revised Edition, Urbana, Illinois: University of Illinois Press.
Knowles, W., and Masidlover, M. (1982) *Derbyshire Language Scheme*, Derbyshire County Council.
Koluchova, J. (1972) Severe deprivation in twins: a case study. *Journal of Child Psychology and Psychiatry* **13** (2), pp. 107–114.
Koluchova, J. (1976) The further development of twins after severe and prolonged deprivation: a second report. *Journal of Child Psychology and Psychiatry* **17** (3), pp. 181–188.
Kratochwill, T. (1981) *Selective Mutism: Implications for Research Treatment*, New Jersey: Lawrence Erlbaum Associates.

Labov, W. (1970) 'The logic of non-standard English' in F. Williams (ed.) *Language and Poverty*, Chicago: Markham Press.
Locke, A. (1985) *Living Language*, Windsor: NFER-Nelson.
Lonton, A., and Halliday, P. (forthcoming) *Physically Disabled Children*, London: Cassell.
Lowe, M., and Costello, A. J. (1976) *The Symbolic Play Test*, Windsor: NFER-Nelson.
Lunzer, E., and Gardner, K. (eds) (1979) *The Effective Use of Reading*, London: Heinemann (For the Schools Council).
Lunzer, E., and Gardner, K. (1984) *Learning from the Written Word*, Edinburgh: Oliver and Boyd (For the Schools Council).
Luria, A. R. (1961) *The Role of Speech in the Regulation of Normal and Abnormal Behaviour*, Oxford: Pergamon Press.

MacKay, G. F. (ed.) (1986) *The Named Person*, Glasgow: Jordanhill College Sales and Publications.
Mackay, D., Thompson, B., and Schaub, P. (1970) *Breakthrough to Literacy*, London: Longman.
McNeill, D. (1966) 'Developmental linguistics' in F. Smith and G. A. Miller (eds) *The Genesis of Language*, Cambridge, Massachusetts: MIT Press, pp. 15–84.
Manning, K., and Sharp, A. (1977) *Structuring Play in the Early Years at School*, London: Ward Lock Educational.

Markides, A. (1970) The speech of deaf and partially hearing children with special reference to factors affecting intelligibility. *British Journal of Disorders of Communication*, 5, pp. 126–140.

Marsh, G., Friedman, M., Welch, V., and Desberg, P. (1980) 'The development of strategies in spelling' in U. Frith (ed.) *Cognitive Processes in Spelling*, London: Academic Press, pp. 339–353.

Meadow, K. P. (1980) *Deafness and Child Development*, London: Edward Arnold.

Meek, M. (1982) *Learning to Read*, London: The Bodley Head.

Miller, G. A. (1951) *Language and Communication*, New York: McGraw-Hill.

Miller, J. F., and Marriner, N. (1986) Language intervention software: myth or reality. *Child Language Teaching and Therapy* 2 (1), pp. 85–95.

Mills, A. E. (1983) 'Acquisition of speech sounds in the visually-handicapped child' in A. E. Mills (ed.) *Language Acquisition in the Blind Child: Normal and Deficient*, London: Croom Helm, pp. 46–56.

Mitchell, D. (1976) 'Parent–child interaction in the mentally handicapped' in P. Berry (ed.) *Language and Communication in the Mentally Handicapped*, London: Edward Arnold, pp. 161–183.

Mittler, P. (1971) *The Study of Twins*, Harmondsworth: Penguin Books.

Moon, C. (ed.) (1985) *Practical Ways to Teach Reading*, London: Ward Lock Educational.

Moore, T. E. (ed.) (1973) *Cognitive Development and the Acquisition of Language*, London: Academic Press.

Morley, M. (1965) *The Development and Disorders of Speech in Childhood* 2nd edn, London: Churchill Livingstone.

Müller, D. J. (1980) 'A critical evaluation of learning techniques in language therapy' in F. M. Jones (ed.) *Language Disability in Children*, Lancaster: MTP, pp. 1–14.

Müller, D. J. (ed.) (1984) *Remediating Children's Language: Behavioural and Naturalistic Approaches*, Beckenham, Kent: Croom Helm.

Murphy, K. P. (1976) 'Communication for hearing-handicapped people in the United Kingdom and the Republic of Ireland' in H. H. Oyer (ed.) *Communication for the Hearing Handicapped: An International Perspective*, Baltimore: University Park Press, pp. 155–222.

Nelson, K. (1973) Structure and strategy in learning to talk. *Monographs of the Society for Research in Child Development*, No. 38.

Newton, M. J., and Thomson, M. E. (1976) *Aston Index*, Wisbech, Cambridgeshire: LDA.

Northern, J. L., and Downs, M. P. (1978) *Hearing in Childhood*, Baltimore: Williams and Wilkins.

Quigley, S. P., and Kretschmer, R. E. (1982) *The Education of Deaf Children*, London: Edward Arnold.

Raban, B. (1985) (ed.) *Practical Ways to Teach Writing*, London: Ward Lock Educational.

Reynell, J. (1969) A developmental approach to language disorders. *British Journal of Disorders of Communication* 4, pp. 33–40.

Reynell, J. (1977) *Reynell Developmental Language Scales* (Revised), Windsor: NFER.

Richman, N., Stevenson, J. E., and Graham, P. J. (1982) *Pre-school to School: A Behavioural Study*, London: Academic Press.

Robertson, I. (1980) *Language Across the Curriculum: Four Case Studies*, London: Methuen. (For the Schools Council.)

Rogers-Warren, A. K., Warren, S. F., and Baer, D. M. (1983) 'Interactional basis of language learning' in K. T. Kernan (ed.) *Environments and Behavior – The Adaptation of Mentally Retarded Persons*, Baltimore: University Park Press.

Rosen, C. (1971) 'Object lesson' in A. Jones and J. Mulford (eds) *Children Using Language*, London: Oxford University Press, pp. 13–25.

Rushby, N. J. (1979) *An Introduction to Educational Computing*, Beckenham, Kent: Croom Helm.

Rutherford, D. (1977) 'Speech and language disorders and minimal brain damage' in J. G. Millichap (ed.) *Learning Disabilities and Related Disorders*, London: Year Book Medical Publishers, pp. 45–50.

Rutter, M. (1980) 'Language training with autistic children: how does it work and what does it achieve?' in L. A. Hersov, and M. Berger (eds) *Language and Language Disorders in Childhood*. Book supplement to the *Journal of Child Psychology and Psychiatry*, 2, Oxford: Pergamon Press, pp. 147–172.

Rutter, M., and Madge, N. (1976) *Cycles of Disadvantage: A Review of Research*, Heinemann: London.

Rutter, M., and Martin, J. A. M. (eds) (1972) *The Child with Delayed Speech*, Clinics in Developmental Medicine (43), London: Heinemann Medical Books.

Rutter, M., Tizard, J., and Whitmore, K. (1970) *Education, Health and Behaviour*, London: Longman.

Schaffer, R. (1977) *Mothering*, London: Fontana.

Schiff, N. B., and Ventry, I. M. (1976) Communication problems in hearing children of deaf parents. *Journal of Speech and Hearing Research* **41** (3), pp. 100–107.

Silva, P. A., McGee, R., and Williams, S. M. (1983) Developmental language delay from 3 to 7 years and its significance for low intelligence and reading difficulties at age 7. *Developmental Medicine and Child Neurology*, **25**, pp. 783–793.

Skuse, D. (1984) Extreme deprivation in early childhood II: Theoretical issues and a comparative review. *Journal of Child Psychology and Psychiatry* **25** (4), pp. 543–572.

Smith, E. B., Goodman, K. S., and Meredith, R. (1976) *Language and Thinking in School* 2nd edn, New York: Holt, Rinehart and Winston.

Smith, F. (1978) *Reading*, Cambridge: Cambridge University Press.

Snow, C. E., and Ferguson, C. A. (eds) (1977) *Talking to Children: Language Input and Acquisition*, Cambridge University Press: Cambridge.

Snowling, M. (1980) The development of grapheme–phoneme correspondence in normal and dyslexic readers. *Journal of Experimental Child Psychology*, **29**, 294–305.

Snowling, M. J. (ed.) (1985) *Children's Written Language Difficulties*, Windsor: NFER-Nelson.
Söderbergh, R. (1985) Early reading with deaf children. *Prospects* **XV** (1), pp. 77–85.
Somerset Education Authority (1978) *Ways and Means*, Basingstoke: Globe Education.

Thomas, B., Gaskin, S., and Herriot, P. (1979) *Jim's People*, St. Albans: Hart-Davis Educational.
Thomas, G. (1985) Extra people in the classroom: a key to integration? *Educational and Child Psychology* **2** (3), pp. 102–107.
Tizard, B., and Hughes, M. (1984) *Young Children Learning: Talking and Thinking at Home and at School*, London: Fontana.
Tough, J. (1976) *Listening to Children Talking*, London: Ward Lock Educational.
Tough, J. (1977) *Talking and Learning: A Guide to Fostering Communication Skills in Nursery and Infant Schools*, London: Ward Lock Educational (For the Schools Council).
Trevarthen, C. (1979) 'Communication and co-operation in early infancy: a description of primary intersubjectivity' in M. Bullowa (ed.) *Before Speech: The Beginnings of Human Communication*, Cambridge: Cambridge University Press.
Tumin, W. (1978) Parents' views. *Education Today*, Summer.

Van Uden, A. (1977) *A World of Language for Deaf Children, Part I: Basic Principles. A Maternal Reflective Method*, The Netherlands: Swets and Zeitlinger.
Vellutino, F. R. (1979) *Dyslexia: Theory and Research*, Cambridge, Massachusetts: MIT Press.
Vygotsky, L. S. (1962) *Thought and Language*, Cambridge, Massachusetts: MIT Press.

Ward, A. (1985) *Scots Law and the Mentally Handicapped*, Glasgow: Scottish Society for the Mentally Handicapped.
Webster, A. (1985a) Deafness and reading I: children with conductive hearing losses. *Remedial Education*, **20** (2) pp. 68–71.
Webster, A. (1985b) Deafness and reading II: children with severe hearing losses. *Remedial Education*, **20** (3) pp. 123–128.
Webster, A. (1986a) *Deafness, Development and Literacy*, London: Methuen.
Webster, A. (1986b) Update: the implications of conductive hearing loss in childhood. *Association of Child Psychology and Psychiatry: Newsletter*, **8** (3) pp. 4–14.
Webster, A., and Ellwood, J. (1985) *The Hearing-impaired Child in the Ordinary School*, Beckenham, Kent: Croom Helm.
Webster, A., Wood, D. J., and Griffiths, A. J. (1981) Reading retardation or linguistic deficit? I: interpreting reading test performances of hearing-impaired adolescents. *Journal of Research in Reading*, **4** (2) pp. 136–147.
Wells, G. (1981) *Learning through Interaction*, Cambridge: Cambridge University Press.
Wells, G. (1985) *Language, Learning and Education*, Windsor: NFER-Nelson.

White, M., and East, K. (1981) Selecting objectives in language. *Remedial Education* **16** (4), pp. 171–178.

Wing, L. (1976) (ed.) *Early Childhood Autism* 2nd edn, Oxford: Pergamon Press.

Wood, D. J., McMahon, L., and Cranstoun, Y. (1980) *Working with Under Fives*, London: Grant McIntyre.

Wood, D. J., Griffiths, A. J., and Webster, A. (1981) Reading retardation or linguistic deficit? II: test-answering strategies in hearing and hearing-impaired school children. *Journal of Research in Reading* **4** (2), pp. 148–157.

Wood, D. J., Wood, H. A., Griffiths, A. J., and Howarth, C. I. (1986) *Teaching and Talking with Deaf Children*, London: John Wiley and Sons.

Wood, H. A., and Wood, D. J. (1984) An experimental evaluation of the effects of five styles of teacher conversation on the language of hearing-impaired children. *Journal of Child Psychology and Psychiatry*, **25**, pp. 45–62.

Wray, D. (1985) *Teaching Information Skills through Project Work*, Sevenoaks: Hodder and Stoughton.

Name Index*

*DES reports are listed in the Subject Index, under the name of the chairperson.

Subject Index*

*T after a page number indicates a table, F a figure.

WM475.